KIM'S PROMISE

KIM'S PROMISE
A Prince on a Dangerous Mission

Susan Brandt

BROWN
DOG
BOOKS

Published under licence by Brown Dog Books and
The Self-Publishing Partnership Ltd, 10b Greenway Farm, Bath Rd,
Wick, nr. Bath BS30 5RL, UK

www.selfpublishingpartnership.co.uk

ISBN printed book: 978-1-83952-814-9

Cover design by Susan Brandt
Internal design by Andrew Easton

Printed and bound in the UK

This book is printed on FSC® certified paper

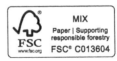

Thanks to some of my early readers,
both young and older:
Sophia, Julius, Alex, Philip, Olivia,
Elisabeth, Sid and Nick

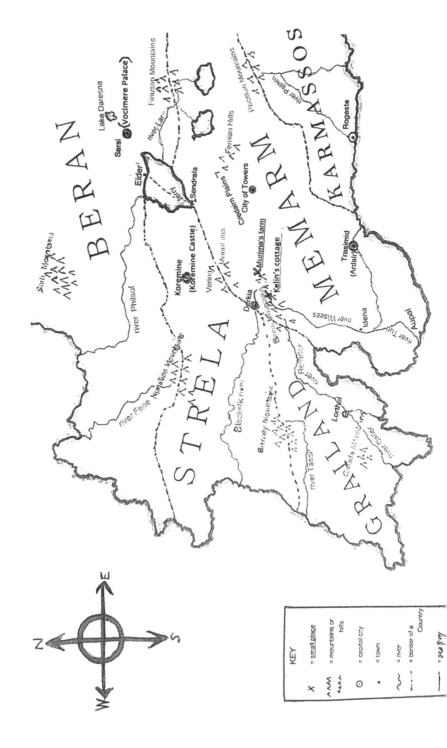

CONTENTS

OPENING
THE QUARREL

A storm was raging in the hills of Strela, where the ancient Koremine Castle stood. The castle was situated in a slight dip amongst the green, rolling hills of the countryside and sounds blew and cackled around it, creating forgotten noises and disturbances in the night. Voices seemed to emanate from everywhere; or were these sounds only created by the searing wind?

In the servants' quarters of the castle, with the rain beating down outside, a few people were clearing up. Balquin was gathering the last bits of washing up from the table and the side dressers to take to the scullery and Sela was giving the great wooden tabletop a scrub with salt. Mira was scraping the remains of a delicious fish pie into a bowl to put into the larder for tomorrow's lunch and Jovo was sweeping the floor ready to wash it over with a mop.

"Have you seen the mess Cook made with the pudding?" Sela joked with Jovo, tipping more salt onto the table as she scrubbed.

"If it had been one of us, we'd have been for it," he responded quickly and, laughing, picked up some of the bits up with a cloth, out of the way of Sela's scrubbing.

"What's that?" Sela jumped and stopped the noisy scrubbing brush.

"Ssh …" Balquin whispered, also stopped in his tracks with the broom.

A crash of thunder, silence, then screaming and shouting from the tower at the top of the narrow, winding stairs which led from the kitchens up to a section of the royal quarters: the old library, to be exact.

"What's happening?" Sela whispered.

"Where's the noise coming from?" Jovo intervened.

"It sounds like a quarrel upstairs!"

They stood about listening.

"From the tower…" Mira said quietly.

"The library," Jovo gasped.

"I can't understand a word of it," ventured Balquin, as the bashing rain and thunder permeated everywhere.

"How does the sound get down here? It sounds all distorted," Jovo added.

The tower was where the noise was coming from. And it was a quarrel. But they couldn't actually hear the words, for the echoing sounds were distorted by the storm. Only, all four of the kitchen staff still remaining in the kitchens that night knew that something terrible was happening in that turret, way above them.

"How dare you?" came the shrill and anguished voice of Queen Porla. And then: "I never thought it possible! … What sons have I given birth to?"

Cook had come in from the scullery, the towel still in her hands.

"What on earth is that to-do up there? Can I hear

shouting or is it just the wind and thunder? Sounds as if it's coming from the top!"

"They're having a quarrel," Jovo answered, as they all stopped to listen again.

The words, "Ashamed of you!" came again from the queen.

And then: "We had to do this!" from one of the princes.

"Sounds like Prince Demble," said Balquin.

"And you, their father!" from the distraught queen again and, in response from King Strearn: "Porla! You can't say ..." A deep voice tapering off as the wind blew it away.

The rest was a muddle of echoing sounds which managed to escape while the wind and the rain beat down all around them and the thunder gave intermittent blasts.

"You go up and listen." Sela eyed Balquin coyly. "Tell us what they're all screaming about."

"Me? No, definitely not!" retorted Balquin.

"Oh, please, Balquin! I really want to know what it's all about." She eyed Balquin cheekily, as Cook shook her head in disapproval and went back towards the pantry.

"I'll give you a kiss if you do ..." Sela went on. "It's only one flight of stairs."

Now, Sela was a very pretty girl and this needed serious thought. Yes, but the steep tower steps went on and on; you couldn't really call it *one flight of stairs!* Even in the daytime those stone steps were a challenge. On the other hand, a kiss from Sela – wouldn't that be worth it, despite the twisting steps, or the sounds now going around and around?

"What do you think Jovo? A kiss from Sela?" The two boys laughed.

"It's only one flight of steps!" repeated Sela.

"Yes, but it winds on and on and the steps are steep and narrow!" Balquin wasn't yet decided. He knew how dark it was on those winding stairs, how cold and dank. "Ok, I'll do it. But promise: a kiss afterwards, Sela…"

"When you tell me what all the trouble's about, yes," she said solemnly. "I promise."

"Good." And Balquin turned and quickly made his way towards the nearby steps which would take him to the top of the turret above them. No-one liked having to go up these cold, narrow steps even in the daytime. At night, it was lit only with a few shielded, flickering candles.

At this moment the sounds, both of thunder and the quarrel, were bouncing around all over the place, as Balquin tried with difficulty to run up the steps two at a time. My God, what a noise! Voices suddenly seemed to pitch towards him:

"Murderers!" the queen screamed. "How can I bear …" and the rest was lost again, in a clap of thunder.

As Balquin got nearer the top, he slowed down. Should he really be doing this? What if he heard things that were private and intended only for the royal family? He suddenly felt afraid. But then, he thought, what about that kiss? It would surely be worth it! Another thought came to him: what if he were discovered? No, he could hide in that utility cubby-hole they had up there, behind the thick curtain; that was right next to the library. He would hear everything from there.

The thunder seemed to have died down a bit, but wind was still whistling around the turret, piercing Balquin's ears as he reached the top. He found the cubby hole and got behind its thick curtain, feeling a bit safer. But what was he hearing now?

"… Poisoned them!" came from the screaming queen.

"Well of course we didn't mean to do that!" retorted her eldest son, Prince Demble. "It just happened. We couldn't help it."

"They had to get the money from somewhere!" came the deep voice of the king.

"Oh, my God …" the queen wailed. And the sound was drowned out by the gusts of wind buffeting the turret.

Balquin stood there in the dark, behind the thick velvet curtain, waiting to hear exactly what they were shouting about. He suddenly needed to know very precisely. He waited and listened; and what he heard sent more than shivers down his spine.

"What you did was fail to stop the people being killed! Poisoned …!" The queen's voice faded and came back again: "You're murderers! My sons are …" and a thunderclap drowned out the sounds again.

A few more moments of listening to the verbal battle of the king, the queen and the two princes, and Balquin was shaking. He was shaking with fear. He was hearing things now he'd never dreamt of and he stood there transfixed and in shock.

What was clear to him was that Queen Porla had discovered something horrible, something that would put the entire family to shame, that the two princes had done with the assistance, or leadership even, of their cold, calculating father, King Strearn.

Balquin was shaking both with the terror of what he had heard and the sudden realisation that if one of them came out of the library now, they would easily find him hiding in the cubby-hole.

After what seemed like an age, Balquin managed to get himself out of the cubby-hole, clattering into a bucket on his way out, which was luckily drowned out by a gust of wind, and grope along the landing towards the steep stone steps which would take him back to the kitchens. There was no thought of Sela or of kisses now. He grabbed hold of the rail, clutching at it hard because he felt shaky and knew that he could fall at any time: it was a long way down.

In the kitchens, Sela, Jovo and Mira joked together.

"We'll soon know all about it!" said Mira. "We'll know why she's screaming up there!"

"And Balquin will get that kiss from Sela," quipped Jovo.

"All right, all right … I know. But it's worth it to find out, isn't it?" Sela pleaded.

Balquin was reaching the bottom of the steps now. He was sweating and shivering at the same time. And he felt faint. The kiss was forgotten, the questions were more like: would he be able to get to the kitchen and what would he tell them?

At the door of the kitchen, he staggered forward and then collapsed onto the floor.

"What's the matter?" Sela exclaimed. "Are you alright?"

"What's happened?" Jovo ran to him. "Oh my God! What's happened?"

"Did someone hurt you?"

"No, I'm alright." But Balquin was visibly in shock and white as a sheet.

"I'll get Cook," said Mira, distressed, and she ran to the pantry.

A moment later Cook came in. "Now, what's all this about?" she said sternly.

"It's my fault," said Sela. "I dared him to go up and listen to what they were all screaming about."

"I doubt if the poor boy is in any state to tell you that," said Cook, clearly put out to see one of her kitchen staff sitting on the half-washed floor in such a state. "What's the matter with the boy? Quick, get some elderflowers and chamomile. That will calm him. Run, child!"

Sela, followed closely by Mira, ran out towards the pantry where they kept all the herbs, as Jovo attempted to hold his friend in a sitting position on the floor.

"Are you all right there? You've given us a fright. What on earth were they saying up there?" But Balquin just shook his head in silence.

The two girls came back with the tea they had made.

"Did you put honey into it? He's had a shock. He needs something sweet!"

"Yes, we did," answered Sela.

Cook took the mug of tea from Sela and watched as Balquin drank it sip by sip. "What's this all about?" asked Cook, sternly.

"It was me," said Sela. "I dared him," Sela repeated, ashamed.

"What *were* they saying up there?" Jovo questioned Balquin again. "Was it the whole family?"

"Please don't ask me … its' terrible …" Balquin said in anguish. "I don't want to … ever speak of it! I want to forget everything I heard!"

"Listen, it's quieter now …" Sela put in. They were all silent for a moment.

"It's just that the thunder is further away …" Jovo answered.

"No. They've stopped shouting and screaming."

"I can still hear the queen sobbing," responded Mira.

"And the princes talking," went on Jovo

"Finish that up, my dear," said Cook kindly to Balquin, "and you, Jovo, take him to his room and make sure he gets into bed. And that's enough eavesdropping for one night! He's in no fit state to walk on his own or to talk to you; but he'll probably be better in the morning."

So Jovo pulled Balquin up from the floor and the two staggered out of the kitchen, up a nearby short flight of stairs.

"What happened, Balquin?" Jovo asked as they moved towards their joint bedroom. "You've gone completely white, you know."

"Have I?" Balquin said, weakly.

"What did they say? Did they see you?"

"No. Luckily."

"What did they say that's made you like this?"

"I can't tell you … I can't tell you. It's so horrible …"

"My God. You poor thing. I hope those herbs will help you." Jovo, upset by his friend's predicament, got Balquin into bed and tucked him up tightly. "Maybe a good sleep will make you feel better."

* * *

The next day, they were all shelling peas and peeling potatoes in the kitchen.

"How are you feeling?" Sela asked Balquin after a moment.

"I'm all right," he answered without looking at her, continuing the peeling.

At that moment, Mira came running in from outside. "Have you heard?" she said.

"Heard what?" answered Sela.

"Queen Porla!"

"What about her?" Sela stopped shelling her peas.

"She's been found dead! There's going to be one week of mourning for the whole country."

Balquin had stopped peeling potatoes.

"How did she die?" he asked, staring at Mira

"They said she died of food poisoning, but there's talk that she took her own life."

"Took her own life?" repeated Balquin.

"Why would she do that?" questioned Sela.

"Shame ..." said Balquin quietly. Then he went on. "Or someone else could have taken it ..."

"Why would they?" emitted Sela. "What do you mean, Balquin?"

9

"Work that out for yourself," he muttered as Jovo came into the kitchen.

"You're all looking glum."

"Didn't you hear?" asked Sela.

"Hear what?"

"About Queen Porla. She died ..." Sela answered.

"There's a week of mourning," Mira moaned. "It's pretty shocking ... I suppose that means extra work for us. The wake, the funeral. All that."

"How did she die?" asked Jovo.

"Food poisoning, they say ..."

"Oh well, it must be our fault, then!" Mira put in again with irritation. "Whenever things go wrong, the servants are to blame ..."

Balquin, looking down at the floor, muttered again, "They know perfectly well it wasn't our fault."

"What do you mean?" Jovo challenged.

"Nothing ... nothing. I don't mean anything really." And Balquin turned back to peeling potatoes in silence. The others looked at each other.

"And you still won't tell us what you heard?" persisted Jovo. But Balquin, remained silent. The others could see him shaking slightly.

Only Balquin's mind was racing; had she taken her own life, or was it murder? And what if someone from the court had found out that there had been a listener to that quarrel? What if Balquin's own life was in danger?

These thoughts swirled around his head and at night he was unable to sleep as, in their shared room, Jovo listened to Balquin tossing and turning.

The following breakfast, Balquin hardly spoke at all.

"He's really worried," Jovo said to the girls when Balquin was out of the room. "He's frightened."

And the next morning, Balquin was found not to be in his bed. His meagre belongings were missing and Jovo was frantic.

"Where could he be?" Sela asked as they sat at the large kitchen table.

"Why would he just disappear?" asked Cook.

"I think he thought something might happen to him …" Jovo let out.

"Was it anything to do with what he heard in the tower?"

But no-one could answer.

Days later, Mira had more bad news about the court activities from one of the stable boys.

"The king is sending soldiers to find one of the kitchen boys who is suspected of being a spy."

They now went about their chores in the kitchen in silence; none of them wanted to be thought guilty of eavesdropping. But after three months, the soldiers told the king that the kitchen boy must have died of hunger or drowned in the nearby lake, because they couldn't find him anywhere.

None of them at that time realised the effects the queen's death and the importance of Balquin's disappearance would have on the whole country. But that was to be in the future, when Prince Demble was the king and his son, Prince Kim, was sent by his mother, Queen Donata, on a fiendishly difficult errand.

Chapter 1
HIDE AND SEEK

TEN YEARS LATER

King Strearn had died some years ago and King Demble now ruled the beautiful country of Strela, with its rolling hills and mountains to the north. He and his wife, Queen Donata, with their young family, Prince Kim, who was nine, and Princess Pala, aged six, had all come to visit the Beran royal family in the bright, lively city of Sarsi, north of Strela, in the country of Beran. Beran was ruled by King Ambab and his wife, Queen Flura, with their two daughters, Princess Sagesse, who was seven, and Princess Effie aged five.

As they entered the great hall of Vocimere Palace, the large home of the Beran royal family set on the northern edge of Sarsi, the two kings made their way up the wide, carpeted stairs together, discussing seriously:

"I think we must work to keep the robbers away," King Ambab said quietly to King Demble. This was an ongoing problem – robbers and brigands both at the borders and inside the country. It was something King Ambab had been working on for years, but he needed to work together with the neighbouring country, Strela, to have some success.

"They've done untold damage in our country. It makes me furious!" King Demble replied. "Have you had robbers recently?"

"Oh yes, we have! I even have ministers working on the problem. At last, I think they are starting to get somewhere …"

The two kings commiserated as they went up, while Queen Donata and Queen Flura talked about the state of the gardens and how to educate their children properly, as well as the fact that Queen Flura had arranged for tea to be taken outside, under the veranda.

As they moved towards the garden, Queen Donata turned to Kim and Pala.

"Why don't you go off and play?" Then, turning to Queen Flura, said, "is that all right?"

"A very good idea," Queen Flura replied. "We can have tea under the veranda and have a nice chat." She was happy to have this rare visit from the neighbouring royals and not be fussing as much as she so often did. "Off you go!" she said, turning to the children. "And remember, the garden is very big, so don't get lost!" She laughed and turned back to Queen Donata, taking her arm and leading her towards the veranda as the children made their way into the garden.

Kim smiled at Sagesse. He had always liked her and felt she was a kindred spirit – perhaps because they were both the eldest child of a family. He somehow knew that being part of his family was special but he didn't know how or why – and, because he had never known anything else, it was really completely normal to him. And yet he had this vague feeling that something was very wrong, and that feeling gave him a sense of great loneliness which he didn't like, so he always put it out of his mind as quickly as he could. But being with Sagesse took away that sense of loneliness, even though they didn't see each other often.

Now, Pala turned to her older brother: "I love it when we come here, don't you? Father doesn't ever tell us off in front of King Ambab, does he?" Kim laughed as Pala went on loudly: "Can we play hide and seek? It's so exciting here!"

They all agreed and the four children trouped into the back part of the great garden which surrounded the palace; here it was wilder, less pruned and sculpted than the parts near to the veranda.

"I'll hide," said Kim. "You all have to find me. Close your eyes and count to one hundred."

There was no questioning him and the girls closed their eyes and started to count as Kim rushed off, then changed direction and ran towards trees in the darker, more closely wooded area, near the back part of the garden.

Surrounding these palace gardens there were high walls. At the front, by the great main gateway and entrance, the gardens were sculpted lawns and banks of colourful flowers. But at the back of the palace it was wilder: grass, which gave way to a wooded area, with beautiful trees of all kinds where the children could play and, beyond that, towards the outer wall, a dark, mossy area.

It was here that Prince Kim found the most perfect place to hide: a wide and large hollow oak tree, which had some of its roots growing inside, allowing him to sit there comfortably. Having climbed into the tree, he now half-sat, half-lay on a root in the hollow, picking at a stick as he waited for the girls to find him.

But it seemed only minutes later Sagesse was there. "I've found you!" she laughed and crowded inside the oak with Kim.

"Isn't it cosy in here? I've been here before," said Sagesse. "But it's better with two – and I've never shown Effie."

"Why not?" Kim was quite impressed that she had found his wonderful hiding place so quickly.

"She would probably be scared," said Sagesse seriously.

"Scared? How ridiculous! Why?"

"She's scared of a lot of things. Spiders, for one thing. She wouldn't dare come near this oak tree!" They looked around the inside of this dank, dark tree. "Are you scared of anything?"

"Well …" He thought for a moment. "The thing that scares me most – but you mustn't tell – is when my father loses his temper. It used to frighten me more, but I still am scared sometimes. My father," said Kim sadly, "can get into a temper about anything if things aren't just as *he* wants them …"

"Oh dear … Mother is a bit like that. But sometimes Father just tells her off quietly and she stops."

"I wish King Ambab could come and do that with my father!" They laughed for a moment.

"Can you smell the flowers?" asked Sagesse suddenly. "I can smell the flowers outside. I'm going to pick some." She eased herself carefully out of the tree, then bent down to smell the little flowers that grew around it.

"Don't let them see you ..." cautioned Kim.

Sagesse looked around. "They've gone the other side of the palace." She laughed. "And there are nuts here. The squirrels must have put them down." She picked up a few, took a stone, broke their shells and ate them. "Here. Try them. Hazelnuts." Sagesse broke a few more, came back to the oak tree and put a few nuts into Kim's hand. As he ate them Sagesse started to sing very quietly: *"I had a little nut tree, nothing would it bear, but a silver nutmeg and a golden pear. The king of Spain's daughter came to visit me. And all because of my little nut tree ..."*

Kim looked thoughtful. "I've got a sad song. Shall I sing it?"

Sagesse nodded, with her finger to her lips. So, very quietly, Kim sang his sad song, which went something like this: *"How sad I am, how sad I am, my love is a long way away. How sad I am, how sad I am, I wish I could be near to say: how glad I am, how glad I am, that we are together this day."*

They sat inside the tree talking seriously and quietly for a long time. "You won't tell my father what I said?" said Kim. "He would call me a baby."

"I won't tell your father," Sagesse said solemnly.

"And ..." Kim hesitated a moment. "If you ever need me for anything please ask me or call on me and I will come ... if I can."

"Thank you. And I will do the same for you."

They both gave a laugh and went on laughing and joking until, suddenly, both Effie and Pala were there.

"At last! We've found you!" they shouted with relief.

"We couldn't find you …" wailed Effie, the youngest of the four. "I thought you had really got lost and disappeared."

"Come on," said Sagesse. "Maybe there's some tea and cakes. I'm hungry." And they all trouped back to the Palace.

* * *

As he got older, Kim found himself having more and more arguments with his father and it was a relief when, aged fifteen and tall for his age, Queen Donata sent him away on his horse, Plarus, to deliver a package to her old home in the north of Strela, at the foothills of the Klandin Mountains.

He was delighted with this task and after delivering the package, Kim rode on further, to visit Sagesse and her family to stay for a few days, where he had some nice conversations with King Ambab and was able to play a few sports – tennis and volleyball, amongst them – with Sagesse.

But a few days before Kim's arrival from the Klandin Mountains, Sagesse's parents had been in the large sitting room, drinking tea, having a rather heated conversation about their daughter's future: they had discussed a betrothal.

"Of course, she's only thirteen and she won't marry

until she's seventeen, but I do think a long engagement is a good thing so that they can get to know each other before marriage," Queen Flura stated firmly. She had worked out her arguments before broaching the subject with King Ambab because she knew Prince Kim was coming soon and she needed to make her feelings clear. She knew King Ambab might not like what she had to say.

"I don't disagree with you, my dear," answered King Ambab. "But it is important that she likes the person, isn't it? It's the characters of the suitors that matters – whether they are good people or not – that kind of thing. Young Kim would make a good husband for her, I think. And they get on very well."

"I am not keen on him despite his good looks." Queen Flura turned away from her husband in pique. "You remember that time they hid in the tree. For hours! Then they came out covered in moss, with their clothes terribly spoilt! Sagesse's beautiful dress was quite muddy! Effie and Pala were frantic looking for them. And that young Kim didn't seem to notice at all. No, he'll probably grow up to be just like his father, bossy, belligerent, egotistic and – so I've heard – with quite a temper."

"Well, that may be King Demble; it doesn't mean his son is the same."

"He's not on the list of suitors! He's rather too independent-minded for my taste."

"I should think a lot of it depends on Sagesse's ideas, doesn't it?" Ambab said quietly. "I'm sure Sagesse is fond of him."

"How can you know that?"

"I don't *know* it. I sense it in her. I know my own daughter."

Ambab got up from his chair and went to the bookshelf in this spacious but comfortable room to avoid Queen Flura's silent fury. As if *she* didn't know her own daughters! - she thought. She wanted to scream, but instead clutched at the arms of her chair with her nose in the air trying, not very successfully, to show indifference.

But now Prince Kim had come to the palace and as they walked around the garden, Sagesse told him despondently that Queen Flura was talking about planning her betrothal; her mother was going to find a nice, wealthy count perhaps, to be husband and companion to her eldest daughter through her life. Sagesse had been dismayed. "A stranger!" she had said again and again. "Why would I want to marry a stranger?"

Kim was shocked and had no answer for her. Why indeed? he thought. She should be married to someone she knows and loves! But he was unable to voice his anguish at this news and had no way to comfort her.

* * *

When he got back to Koremine Castle, even King Demble noticed that Kim was sad and disconsolate and his father seemed to take pleasure in tormenting him with new strictures about his comings and goings and an insistence that he study what the king wanted, rather than what interested Kim himself.

The quarrels between Kim and the king got louder

and more violent, while at the same time Queen Donata started to absent herself from the family meals, preferring to eat alone in her quarters. Kim knew that his mother hated the quarrels that King Demble thrived on, and she wanted no part of them.

"I don't even want to be king, if it's being like you!" Kim blurted out helplessly one day as his father shouted at him. "Anyway, why does Mother never come down to meals nowadays?"

"Your mother! You want her to defend you, do you? Well – she's not feeling well!"

"What's the matter with her?"

"A headache. She feels sick. I don't know precisely."

"Has the doctor been?"

"Lemina is looking after her."

But Kim found himself clenching his fists in fury, while Pala gave him a long, sad look from across the dinner table. Without warning something had taken hold of Kim. Slamming his fist down onto the table, he got up and ran out, banging the door behind him. Outside, he burst into a silent rage that took him over: he wanted to punch his father down to the floor. He wanted to do all sorts of violent things to him! Why was he in such an explosion of temper? Why did it have to be like that with his father? It was unbearable! And not only that, but he was finding it increasingly difficult to do his studies.

Pala, left alone with her angry father, stayed at the table eating quietly. She knew Kim had been right to get back at their father. The king was always saying Kim was lazy, but she didn't think he was; she knew he worked hard at his studies.

"May I leave the table, Father?" She asked quietly, when she had finished.

"Yes. Yes, you may, dammit!"

Pala ran out of the dining room and burst into tears, running to her room in despair. Why was everything so difficult? She threw herself onto the bed. What could she do?

She felt helpless.

* * *

"How are things going?" Cal, Kim's friend, asked Kim that evening.

"Bad ..." Kim moaned. "My father shouts at me and tells me to study what *he* wants…"

"Oh! How terrible. I don't know how you can bear it. Thank God my father doesn't do that!"

"Well, I've never known any other father, have I? And the fact is, also, I'll have to be king one day," said Kim sadly. He turned to Cal. "What I'd really love to do is to travel. I went up to Beran on my horse, Plarus, to see the royal family there."

"Is that your friend the Princess Sagesse?"

"Yes. But her mother is going to try to get her married off to someone as soon as she can. And the queen doesn't like me much, really. But I was glad to see the countryside and the people in it. There is terrible hardship in the country, you know." He remembered the worn, haggard

21

faces of the farmers and the rags they wore as he travelled his way across the Klandin Mountains on his way to Vocimere Palace.

"Would you ask for money from your father if you went travelling?"

"I'd rather work my way around, doing odd jobs."

"And what does your mother say about that?"

"I haven't told her!" And Kim told Cal about his mother staying away and how silent and sad Pala was: "While I just get into a rage!" he added.

He got back late from Cal's and came in quietly through a side door. As he was coming up the back stairs, he heard two servants talking in one of the rooms. It was Sen, who had been with the royal family since King Demble and Queen Donata had got married and another younger man, whose voice Kim didn't recognise. But what he heard them saying stopped him in his tracks. "The king's ordered the south wing to be completely redecorated and refurbished so that his mistress can live there?" the younger of the two servants was saying.

"How do you know it's for his mistress?" Sen had replied.

"He virtually said so …" answered the other. "He said he was fed up with the queen keeping away from him in her quarters, and he was moving a close lady-friend into the south wing, so that he could have some company."

"What's her name?" asked Sen.

"Drina."

"Well, I don't know!" said Sen. "The queen hasn't said anything to us for a month now. Does she know what's happening?"

Kim had heard enough to make him feel sick. He crept up the stairs and over the wide landing to his room and went quickly to bed. He would talk to his mother in the morning. He knew she never came down to meals now, but this: what did it mean?

The next morning Kim had an early breakfast and then went straight up to see his mother. Despite his shock and dismay at what he had heard the night before, he had been thinking and had made some plans. He knew things were terribly wrong and were affecting everyone badly, especially his mother, but also Pala, who was becoming more and more silent and morose, and himself so often in a rage and fury about his father and about the ruination of the country.

Kim knocked firmly on his mother's door. There was no answer. He knocked again, louder, calling softly: "It's me, Mother …" He waited. "It's me … Kim," he called again. He heard steps. The door was being unlocked from the inside. Eventually it opened slowly and his mother stood there.

He stepped back involuntarily. She had changed. It was more than a week since he'd seen her and she looked different: her hair whiter and her skin pale. Or was he imagining it? She opened the door wider for him. He entered, wondering about the fusty smell.

"How are you?" He kissed her.

"Oh, I don't seem to get much better." She stroked his brow as if he were the one who was ailing. "It's this pain in my head and eyes," she said. "The only thing that helps me is to lie down with a damp cloth over my eyes."

She lay down onto her bed and Kim put the damp cloth over her forehead and eyes, which she removed every so often to talk and to look at him. He drew up a chair.

"Mother," Kim went on, "I overheard something last night …"

"And what was that?"

"It was Sen and one of the other servants, talking."

"What did they say?"

"They were talking about Father – that he's having the south wing refurbished so that … so that … he can move … a lady-friend in there." He was watching his mother to see how she reacted.

"I know about this," she said. "Drina is her name."

"I don't even know who she is …"

"She's a pretty, rather greedy young woman. I'm sorry you had to find out about her like that."

Suddenly, Kim wondered if it was his father's behaviour that was causing his mother's illness.

"Come, tell me what your plans are; I know you've made some plans."

"Well, I'd like to travel and see other countries for myself. Find out how other people live."

The queen looked at Kim lovingly. "I have been waiting for the moment you would want to travel," she said quietly. "I've something I need you to do."

Kim was mystified. How could his mother have known that he wanted to travel? He had said nothing to her about his ideas because he thought she would not approve. But now she was there in front of him, obviously weak and wrapped up in a large gown over bed clothes, saying she had been waiting for this moment.

"I've known for a while that you would travel, just as I know about the task you have to complete."

"Task?"

"Listen carefully." She took his hand. "This is important," she whispered. "A curse has been put onto this family, onto this land indeed. And you're the only person who can get rid of it."

Kim was at a loss. "What curse? What do you mean?"

"If we knew exactly what the curse was, there would be no curse – everything would be clear and in the open. A curse is only powerful when people don't know about it, or what it is. That's when a curse does damage." She paused for breath and then went on: "There was a quarrel which caused the curse, but because neither your father nor your uncle, Prince Callouste, will even acknowledge that the quarrel took place, it remains secret although it has a terrible effect … can affect generations."

"What do you mean? What was the quarrel about?"

"Only one person knows that."

"One person? But how can you know it's a curse?"

"Curses happen when someone bad, someone small-minded and without courage becomes so envious of another person or people that they wish harm on them. In this case something was said during that quarrel, or something came out, that showed that a person or people were seriously harmed. The quarrels you have with your father, how you dislike him, how very angry you get – sometimes for no reason – that is the effect of this curse. Pala is in frequent tears, with tear-stained face and depression although she pretends nothing is wrong; the poverty and starvation in this land even when people work hard. At the same time King Demble cares little for our people; it doesn't register with him that he is responsible if ministers are corrupt and the people starving. In Beran, where King Ambab rules, things are not like this." She stopped for a moment to catch her breath, then went on: "A curse is brought about by terrible envy." Queen Donata stopped and closed her eyes.

"It's funny … I've always thought King Ambab of Beran was a good king," Kim said quietly. "He doesn't get into tempers like father does …"

"You're young," Queen Donata said, "but you can fight. I cannot anymore. One day you'll be in charge of this beautiful country. You will have to do the battling." She had taken off the cloth and was dabbing at the tears falling down her cheeks. "I am tired now," she said. "Come tomorrow. There are still things we need to talk about."

"Of course, Mother. I'll come tomorrow morning."

Kim kissed her and left the room in a daze. What had he heard? What could she mean? Why was she so distraught? A curse? A quarrel which only one person had heard? Was she telling the truth about the corruption of his father's ministers? He had heard about bandits at the borders, but not about corruption within the country and amongst his father's ministers! And yet he did know from his friend, Cal, how people could work extremely hard – as did Cal's parents in their shop – and get little gain from it. Was this part of the curse?

On his way down the stairs, he saw Pala.

"Is mother any better?" she asked him.

"Not really."

"What were you talking about?"

"Oh, I don't know … A quarrel took place a long time ago. Do you know about it?" he asked. Pala shook her head. "I don't think anyone knows. Apparently only one person heard it."

"Was it Mother?"

"No. She doesn't know what the quarrel was about."

"So how does she know it happened?"

"I don't know exactly; she wants me to find out. It's to do with corruption, banditry and a curse that's contaminated the family and the country."

"Oh …" Pala said hesitantly. Then quietly: "I've seen that …"

"Do you know about Drina?" Kim asked suddenly.

"Drina? Who's she?"

"A friend of Father's. He's installing her into the south wing."

Pala looked shocked. "Do you know her?"

"No, but Mother says she's very pretty and very greedy."

"I hope we don't have to see her …" Pala said gravely.

Kim wondered about Drina. Was she important? Perhaps she was, even if only because his mother was upset by her presence.

*   *   *

The next morning, as Kim was going up the stairs to his mother's room, her maid, Lemina, ran down towards him.

"Please sir! Come quickly! … Oh, she's fading sir. Princess Pala is with her. Please hurry!"

They both ran into the queen's quarters and Pala, who was at her mother's bedside, got up and kissed him. "She's been asking for you," Pala said.

"I'm here, Mother." He turned to the maid. "Would you leave us, please?" Lemina gave a little curtsy and left.

"I'll leave also," Pala said. "She wants to speak to you. I'll see you outside." She kissed her mother, then Kim, and left the room.

His mother was lying in bed propped up with cushions, a bowl of water with a damp cloth on the bedside table. She looked even frailer than yesterday, her voice quite weak. "Listen my dear. I haven't told you all of it …"

"All of what, Mother?"

"I told you about the curse, my dear, you must fight to understand it, you must learn to love to fight …"

"Yes, Mother," Kim said, bewildered at the sight of his mother today.

"What I mean is fighting for something. In yourself, for what's good and right, so you can understand things better: the truth and yourself. That's what I mean."

"I think I understand, Mother." He wasn't sure. "But how can I be any use, as it happened before I was born?"

"You can take away this curse, I know you can. But you will need to be determined and brave. And there are

28

two other things." Kim waited. "You will need to keep what you're doing completely secret. If not, it will be much harder for you."

"And what's the other thing?"

"The other thing is that you must find out about this before the *Festival of the King's Rule,* which will install your father on the throne for life and is in November, next year."

"But I don't know what I am trying to find out …" He was still at a loss.

"Find the cause of the quarrel, which I think is also the cause of old Queen Porla's death. Whatever the quarrel was about, it was that quarrel that caused her death and caused the curse." Queen Donata stopped to catch her breath, then looked intently at Kim. "Kim, you need to promise me …"

"Anything, Mother. What do you want me to promise?"

"That you'll do your best to find out about this terrible quarrel and this terrible curse."

"But how do you know about this curse, Mother?"

"I can't list all the things that brought me to an understanding of it, but I've seen the effects of this curse time and again: the cause of Pala's unhappiness and your frequent outbursts of terrible anger. It causes severe illness and starvation in the country and affects badly those we love – and I've been waiting for the day when you'd want to travel. I've always known that you were the one to do it. I need your promise, Kim, that you'll do this."

"Well, yes, I promise. I promise I'll do my best, Mother. Only, I'm not sure how to go about it. Who heard the quarrel? Who knows about it?" Kim wondered for a moment whether he could first go on his travels. But no! His father's important festival: Kim must have his task finished before then.

"There's one man – apart from your father and Callouste, of course – who was a part of this quarrel. I nursed him when he was ill, but he wouldn't say what it was about."

"Well, I'll go and ask him! What's his name? Where is he?"

"He's called Balquin. He's the only person you can talk to about this curse because he's suffered from it; but apart from him, it must remain a secret if you're to be successful. The great difficulty is where to find him. I have no idea where he is. I heard he went to Memarn, or possibly north, to Beran, with papers he'd written about the wrongdoings. Balquin worked here; he was a kitchen boy when he heard the quarrel and you must find him, otherwise the curse will continue on, generation after generation, making it impossible to be free. But you must remember: the one thing Balquin will have done will be to try to erase completely from his memory the horror of what he heard. He left the castle in terror and, if he realises who you are, he is likely to flee from you. That is, unless he trusts you." She lay back with a sigh and caught her breath for a moment.

Kim quickly poured some water for the queen and gave it to her.

"Thank you." She took a sip of the water. "He will trust you if he is sure of you and of who you are." She stopped and lay back. Then she said softly, "I want you to get something out of a drawer ..."

"Where, Mother?"

"The chest of drawers, there." She pointed to the wall. "At the back of the third one down, you'll find a secret compartment covered with a bit of sliding wood."

Kim went to the chest of drawers, counting three down. Feeling carefully amongst scarves and blouses, he slid the piece of wood along and pulled out two little bags. "Are these what you want?" he asked, taking them to her.

She took the little bags and opened them. Inside one, there were two large diamonds; inside the other, two smaller gems. "There used to be three diamonds, all cut the same way. Take one of them with you when you look for Balquin. I gave him the third. The other is for Pala, to give her freedom when she marries. But I think Pala will only marry when you find Balquin and get him to tell you what he knows. I gave one to Balquin after he was brought unconscious to my parents' house and because I was frightened that he'd starve to death. I also showed him how to hide the diamond so robbers wouldn't find it. Give this to him, to compensate him for his troubles and then he will know you've come from me. Sew it into your waistband, the way I've shown you. The two others," she took out the smaller gems, "are for you, in case of need."

"I'll do my best, Mother ... to find Balquin. I promise," said Kim, seriously. "But first, when you're better, I'm going to get somewhere good for you to live and then after that I'll go on my search for him."

Of course, Kim didn't want to acknowledge to himself how ill his mother really was. Also, he didn't really understand the difficulties of what he had promised to do. Even with luck on his side, how could he know the complications entailed in trying to find a person who wanted to disappear? At that moment all he wanted to do was to please his mother and get her well again.

"Thank you, my dear. Find Balquin as quickly as you can. End this frightening curse so that it can't contaminate lives of generations as it has yours and your sister's and mine and many others." And with that she fell back onto the pillows. "Now I feel very tired. Remember what I've said and remember that wherever you are or wherever I am, I will always be in your heart, guiding you …" Then she seemed to fade away.

"No! No, Mother!" Kim rushed out of the room to call Lemina. He shouted down the hall and Lemina ran up the stairs. She quickly reached the bed and felt the queen's head, then put a glass to her lips. Finally, she took her pulse, but there was no sign of life.

* * *

The funeral was three days later and people came to the castle from all around to pay their respects to the much-loved queen. Among the mourners were King Ambab and his family including, of course, Sagesse. Kim longed to speak to her, as he had not seen her since his visit to

Vocimere Palace many months ago and he remembered their childhood pact with fondness.

Eventually, Kim managed to talk to her as she and her family filed past to give their condolences.

"I am going away soon. I have some work in Memarn," said Kim sadly.

Sagesse looked surprised. Memarn was a country well to the south-east of Strela.

"Memarn?" she responded. "What work is that?"

Kim faltered. "I have to find someone who has gone to Memarn. He's got some information I need." He looked at Sagesse intently. "I hope to be back very soon ... so that ..." He stopped. He wanted to say: *So that I am back before your mother has you betrothed to someone else* ... But how could he? He didn't exactly know what it was he felt for Sagesse except closeness. He just knew he wouldn't be able to bear it if she married someone else. Was that love? A feeling of such closeness and understanding that it ruled everything you did?

He understood what his mother had said, that this curse – shaming and unpleasant, causing pain to himself, his mother and Pala, and perhaps the people around them, even the whole country – would continue into the next generation if it were not removed. And the only way to remove this curse was to understand what had happened long ago, the quarrel which had killed Queen Porla. Kim knew that his father, his uncle and grandfather were implicated in it all and this frightened him, but he had no idea how or what it was about.

"I wish you a swift return and a good outcome."

Sagesse sensed the urgency of his mission, though she didn't know why and couldn't ask. She only had the feeling it was dangerous and she wanted him back safe, as soon as possible.

"Thank you, Sagesse," he said and kissed her hand, but his mind was both confused and racing; he was in distress about his mother and anguished as well as fearful about leaving.

That evening, with his friend Cal, he confessed: "She is the most wonderful girl, but I didn't know how to say goodbye. I thought I might never see her again!"

"Why on earth would you think that?" said Cal, taken aback.

"I don't know. Perhaps it was my mother telling me about the urgency, the danger and secrecy of what I have to do to prevent a catastrophe; perhaps it was that, if I'm not back in time, Sagesse's mother might betroth her to some terrible, rich stranger." He looked away from Cal, closing his eyes. "She means too much."

Chapter 2
THE SEARCH

A few days later, King Demble was in another rage, as Kim told him of his plan to go travelling.

"You'll get no money from me for this hare-brained idea!"

"I'll work, on my way ..." Kim faltered and then, shouting, "I'm going to go! I don't care what you think ..."

"And where are you going to go?"

"I don't know!"

"You're just fifteen and you're already a loser," retaliated the king. "Do you think anyone will employ you? Do you really think you'll be fit to be king if you behave like this? You won't get very far at all before you come crawling back." His father gave a sneer and walked out of the dining room where they had been eating supper.

*   *   *

Two weeks later, with a small bag of essentials, Kim went down to the stables. The stable hand had prepared his horse, Plarus, and there stood the handsome, brown stallion, fierce and fast and ready to take Kim anywhere he wanted to go.

"Thank you, Marius." Kim shook the stable boy's hand and walked round to the front of the castle, where Pala was waiting to say goodbye to her brave, fifteen-year-old brother.

"I'll write and let you know where I am and what I am doing," he said to Pala, softly. He knew his departure would be difficult for her but was comforted by the fact that she would soon be away from here, studying with some of her friends. "Don't worry if you don't hear. It might be impossible because I don't want people to know who I am and I might not have the opportunity to write."

"But do write if you can, please ..." Pala embraced him fondly and Kim got up onto his horse and, giving her a wave, rode south, towards Koremine Town, where Cal was waiting for him.

They had arranged that Cal would come part of the way, just to the border of Strela and Grailand to help start Kim on his quest for the kitchen boy. Kim had told Cal about his father and Drina, and they had laughed a little at them and then Kim had become sad because, after all, his mother had died. And then they had agreed that Cal should come part of the way – as long as he didn't ask too many questions.

"I mean, it's not easy to look for someone if you have no real idea where they might be, is it?" Cal had said, wisely.

So now Kim and Cal were riding south, towards the country of Grailand.

"What if he's gone north?" asked Cal.

"My mother mentioned Memarn, so that's where I'm headed first. If I can't find him there, I'll head north to Beran."

Fears and thoughts crowded in on both Kim and Cal as they rode through the beautiful, wooded lanes and green fields of Strela, towards the south. And there was another thing: "I have to find this person soon," Kim asserted. "Within a year or at the very most, before the *Festival of the King's Rule*, because then it will be too late." Kim was glad that Cal didn't question him; Cal knew that he couldn't tell him much. "*And* I have to get back before Queen Flura finds the perfect rich stranger for Sagesse!"

The weather was warm enough for them to sleep outside under the trees, with their horses keeping guard; tomorrow they would find more food. They had slept under the stars once or twice before when they had gone off together for a few days. It would be a bit different when Cal left him; Kim knew that there were often robbers near to the borders. Here though, it was quiet with only a few sheep in the field.

The next day they rode on, waving at the friendly people with their brightly coloured scarves and neckties, singing as they worked in the fields. As evening approached and the sun started to dip, they came near a small farmstead. Maybe they would be able to get some food here.

Getting nearer, they could see that the farm was smaller and poorer than they had thought; the house was in need of repair and the place looked ill-cared for, with two chained dogs barking at them as they went up the path. They knocked loudly and a woman came running towards them from the field.

"What do you want?" she shouted. "Are you from the tax office?"

"No, no," said Kim, perplexed. "We wondered if you've got any work – in exchange for a bit of food and some shelter."

"Work? We've got plenty of work! The boys will be glad of some help, but we haven't got much food. Nobody has enough at the moment with the king's taxes as high as they are. Put the horses in the barn and you can take them some hay later."

"Thank you!" they called and went off to the barn with the horses.

For the rest of the day Kim and Cal spent their energy in the fields, scything wheat and eating a bit of bread and cheese.

"Why is it that these people, who work so hard at something the whole country needs, the whole country depends upon, in fact – the wheat for bread – why do they have to go hungry themselves?" Kim questioned Cal as they lay in some soft straw in the barn that night.

"It's something to do with the taxes, the high payments which go to your father …"

"If I become king, Cal," he said, "I will change it so that poor people don't have to pay so much as the rich, if anything."

The next morning, after being given some bread and cheese for their journey, they left the farmer and his wife and made their way up over the hill and on towards Derkia. There, Kim would again look for work, on his own this time, as Cal was going back to Koremine Town

*   *   *

Derkia, a little, ancient town was just over the border of Grailand, on the main route leading through the Binon Mountains to Memarn. It would be easier to find work here than in the countryside, he thought, and then he could see himself well on the road to what he still hoped was his destination: Trasimid, the great capital of Memarn.

Kim wandered through the narrow streets of Derkia, stopping to dismount Plarus and asking for work at shops and eating places. In one cafe, an old man was sitting outside, smoking a pipe and drinking coffee.

"Excuse me, sir," Kim asked politely, "do you know of any odd jobs going around here by chance?"

The man looked at him blankly, then laughed. "Nah. I don't know of any work going!" And he turned his back on him. But Kim persisted with his search and soon came on someone else.

"Work? Well, I know a tavern on the outskirts, *Trent's Laurels*. They were looking for a worker the other day," the man said and he gave Kim the directions.

Now Kim wound his way through the narrow streets until he arrived at a large tavern, overlooking only a few cottages on the edge of the town. He tied Plarus up outside the tavern and went in. Inside, *Trent's Laurels* was half-filled with people, mainly eating lunch and talking quietly. When he asked, he was directed towards the owner of the tavern, a large, burly, friendly man named Trent.

"My man's had to go off to the country to his sister's who's sick and he doesn't know when he's coming back. So, if you can help for a few weeks, maybe a month with the wine, the beer and the barrels as well as doing some serving at tables, we'd like that. Suit you?"

Trent had seated Kim down on one of the seats at a table. "It's food and board included," Trent added proudly.

"Yes! I'll take it, if you'll have me," laughed Kim, immediately liking the big man and pleased that he would get some food here. "When do I start?"

"Let's set you up with a bit to eat first," said Trent. "Look as if you could do with feeding up a bit. Lamb and potatoes do you?"

Kim smiled brightly and Trent lumbered off to order the promised lamb and came back a moment later with what looked like two small mugs of beer.

"You're not too young for this, are you?" he asked Kim.

"I think I'm allowed, if it's not too strong." Kim laughed.

"No, it's shandy. Got lemon in it." Trent gave a warm gentle laugh. "Travelling then, are you?" he went on.

"Yes, exactly."

"Where from?"

"Strela. The capital, Koremine," Kim answered honestly.

"So, what are you doing in this part of the world – apart from travelling?" Trent asked, taking a drink of his shandy.

"I've been sent by my family" – a bit of truth in this – "to search for my uncle" – a complete lie. "My father needs him to help build a new section to our house. He has some skills, you see." Kim had worked out this story to save any awkward questions. "I won't be able to stay long anyway, because I need to find him."

Trent looked concerned. "Difficult, finding people who've gone off," he said with some strange foresight. "So, you're from Strela?"

"Yes."

"Queen just died there, didn't she?"

Kim was taken aback at Trent's easy reference to his mother. He really *didn't* want people to know he was the Prince of Strela. He wanted to be just an ordinary young man looking for a relative.

"Yeah … my cousin used to work at the palace," invented Kim. "He says she was a lovely person. But I don't know, myself."

"That's what I've heard them say," said the innkeeper. "A truly beautiful person married to a coarse brute, the King of Strela."

"A brute? Is that what they call him over here?" Kim was slightly at a loss.

"Why, what do the Strelans think of him, then?" asked Trent.

"Well, no … I mean, he's tolerated, you know. I've never heard him called a brute, though. What've you heard then?" Kim hoped he was sounding easy-going and unperturbed, when in fact he was nervously bursting with curiosity about what was thought of his family in the country of Grailand.

"There are all sorts of rumours going around about that King Demble," Trent remarked.

"Rumours?" Kim asked as nonchalantly as he could.

"Oh, one was that King Demble and his brother Callouste threatened their mother ..."

"What? How could that be?" Kim paused for a moment, as if he couldn't believe what he was hearing. Then, still pretending disbelief, he added: "When was that?"

"When King Strearn ruled the kingdom."

"Oh. Well, that was long before I was born. I can't imagine King Demble would threaten his mother, would he?" He stopped for a moment, then persisted: "What would he threaten his mother with, anyway?" He wanted to find out anything this kind man knew.

"Don't know. Could be anything really. You never know what people are doing behind closed doors, do you?"

"No. I suppose you don't." Kim took a draught of his shandy. "Do you think maybe they had an argument?"

"Could be, I suppose. Could be worse than an argument; more like a quarrel."

"Yes, now I come to think of it ... I seem to remember some talk of a quarrel in the dim, distant past. I wonder what it could have been!" Kim was still trying to hide his interest in this conversation and not let on his desperation to know what Trent was getting at.

"It was mysterious, I seem to recall," said Trent firmly. "I vaguely remember a person telling me something about a quarrel before she died. The old queen, Porla, that is. Not the one who's just died. It seemed a bit odd at the time though." Trent turned around on his bench towards a man drinking at the next table, behind him. "Edmond," he said, tapping the man's shoulder. "Edmond, you remember who it was told us about the old queen Porla?"

"Who?" said the man, turning in his seat. "How you doing, Trent?" And Edmond, who was thin with dark locks round his ears, gave a laugh and shook Trent's hand.

Trent turned back to Kim, indicating Edmond. "This man, you know, you can ask him anything! A wonderful memory. Though whether politics in Strela is a subject he knows about – we shall see." He gave a chuckle and turned back to Edmond. "Do you remember – many years ago now – someone talked about that old queen Porla when she died, in Strela?"

"Oh, I don't know … Why do you always ask me such difficult questions? That must have been over twenty years ago, Trent!"

"I tell you," Trent turned again to Kim, saying loudly, "his memory is second to none! He'll complain, but then he'll remember the most amazing details." He laughed and then turned back to Edmond. "This young lad's come from Strela where the queen's just died, and I was trying to recall what we heard when old Queen Porla died. I seem to remember it was all a bit strange."

"Oh yes, I can remember that. It was that young chap."

"What young chap?" asked Trent.

"Who told us! He worked for you … You should know! Balkie, I think he called himself. Yes, Balkie, I'm sure of it."

Balkie? Kim gulped. Was this the kitchen boy from Koremine Castle? The name was so similar: *Balkie* …?

"I remember him," Edmond continued. "Clever little chap. Bright as anything. Only with you a short time, wasn't he?"

Trent turned to Kim again. "We get so many in here you know. Strangers and such. I just can't remember them all, can I?"

"No, I suppose not," Kim answered quietly, waiting all ears for any more information that might come.

"A nice young man," Edmond went on. "I remember him. Told us … what did he tell us? Yes, told us about a terrible quarrel and after it the old queen died. That's what he said. Definite. I remember because it was so odd. He wasn't sure whether they had killed her. That was it!"

"My God! That's terrible! 'They' … who do you mean?" Kim let out, now hiding with difficulty his eagerness to know.

"Hullo. I'm Edmond." Edmond had got up and now joined them at their table. He was holding a hand out to Kim.

"How do you do," said Kim, shaking his hand. "Kim. Nice to meet you."

"Likewise," said Edmond, then continued: "I wouldn't know who the 'they' was; the royals I should think. But he used to get very exercised about things, this Balkie person, didn't he Trent? Angry. Remember? He had a fight with a customer once. You remember that, don't you, Trent? Furious he was. Had been a servant there – he said. At Koremine Castle in Strela. Then had to leave because he claimed his life was in danger, would you believe! Well, I'm not sure I actually did believe that!"

Trent took another sip of his shandy and turned to Kim. "King Demble's got a bad reputation here, young man, even if he's liked at home. Whether all that's true, I don't know. Anyway, people love to make up stories, don't they? They'll say anything if it has an effect."

"Do they make up stories?" Kim asked.

There was a silence for a moment as Trent took another draught of his shandy. "People like to make up stories is all I mean. It makes them seem important …"

Edmond was emphatic: "He said he heard the quarrel better than anyone. That was it! That was what he said."

"Did he hear what they said?" Kim gave a little laugh, trying to sound noncommittal.

"I remember he said they destroyed her …" Edmond went on. "I don't know how … Don't you remember him saying this, Trent?"

"Did he?" questioned Trent, obviously not remembering.

"Who? Destroyed who?" Kim asked, trying to hide his excitement.

"Queen Porla. She was dead within a few days." Edmond was nodding seriously.

"That's horrible. But it *is* rather a long time ago, isn't it?"

"Oh, it is. King Demble has been on the throne now for going on nineteen or twenty years, I should think!"

"And the man? What happened to him?" Kim asked casually.

"What man?"

"The servant. You said he was a servant, Ballie, who heard the quarrel. Where did he go?" Kim deliberately got the name a bit wrong.

"Oh, him … He was young. About your age, I shouldn't wonder. Bit older, maybe. I think he said he was going east to Memarn. Don't know what became of him, though. Did you hear, Trent? Someone said, later, he was seen making horseshoes – or was it cartwheels? Anyway, he was working in that end of Trasimid, the capital."

"Trasimid … I see." So, Kim had come in the right direction.

"Striking-looking chap, though."

Just as Kim was marvelling at his luck in meeting with Edmond and his fine memory, a beautiful young girl arrived with some lamb and potatoes.

"This is my daughter, Ondi," Trent said proudly. "She helps me out in the tavern. Ondi, this is Kim, who's going to take over from Nahan until he gets back from his sister's."

Kim shook Ondi's hand formally.

"Hullo. That's good," she said. "We've been struggling

a bit. He should be back after a few weeks, I suppose."

And Kim mulled on the words he had just heard and the amount of searching he still had to do, although now he knew that Trasimid, over the mountains, was the right place to be aiming for.

*   *   *

Kim now started work at the tavern, which he enjoyed. On two occasions he went out with Ondi and a group of friends. The second time they went to a horse race round the main square. The racers raced around the central square at a break-neck speed. Everyone was very excited, shouting and cheering, and something made Kim turn around in his seat. Sitting right behind him, shouting with everyone else, was a woman who looked just like his mother.

"Hurry! Hurry, hurry!" she was shouting and then she got up, turned and walked away. As she did so, with her back to him, Kim realised that she was just an old peasant woman. But it made him think: *I* need to hurry! How will I find Balquin? What am I doing here? If he didn't get a move on to Trasimid soon, Queen Flura might marry Sagesse off before he even had a chance to get back.

The next day, Kim said to Trent: "I have to go on. My father is waiting for my return so that he can get on with building the house," Kim fibbed again. "I'll have to risk the bandits!"

"You might be lucky," said Trent doubtfully. "I sincerely hope you are."

So, within a couple of days Kim had rolled up his belongings, packed the bread, tomatoes and sausage that Ondi had given him and had ridden off towards the Binon Mountains, on the way to Trasimid.

* * *

Meanwhile, in Koremine Castle, Pala was having a difficult time. For one thing, she missed her adored older brother horribly. Without him and with the queen gone, she felt she could not survive here; and her father was becoming more and more silly and infuriating.

"Why don't you wear some pretty clothes for a change? We can have a party. Drina loves parties. Let's have a party!"

"Father, I don't feel like having a party!" Pala was annoyed and tearful. "I feel sad because Kim is away!" Then she turned and, half talking to herself through the tears, mumbled again angrily, "Looking for a stranger – and my mother died not even a month ago!" She faced him again in distress. "Why would I want a party?"

For practically the first time in her life dear, quiet, *"good girl"* Pala had angrily let rip at her insensitive father.

"All right, all right! Calm down. I didn't know you felt so strongly!" King Demble stopped for a moment. "Anyway, who is this stranger he's searching for? Why's he searching for a stranger? I thought he simply wanted to travel."

"Someone who knows something!" Then Pala wished she had kept quiet. "I don't know who it is, anyway," she muttered, under her breath again.

"Knows something? And what is that?"

"I don't know. I have no idea!" she shouted again.

"He never said anything to me about searching for someone!" The king sounded alarmed. And Pala refused to be drawn further on the matter, as he fumed, pacing around the room, trying to sort out what to do.

"Anything to do with my mother, Queen Porla?" the king threw at her.

"I don't know!"

"Because if it is, I need to know about it!" he said, threateningly. "I absolutely need to know about it! I shall have to take measures …!" King Demble sounded seriously intimidating.

"I don't know! I don't know what it's about!" she repeated and, with that, upset and frightened, Pala ran out of the room.

After that, Pala kept quiet. She came down at mealtimes and said little. If Drina was there, Pala said not a word and got up from the table as soon as possible. Often, she stayed with friends, which was a relief and, when she was at the castle, her mother's maid Lemina and Cook kept a good eye on her to make sure she was alright.

One afternoon she went to see Kim's friend, Cal.

"I just wish he would come home soon with all the information he needs," she said to him.

Cal responded gently, realising how upset she was. "I'm sure he'll be back soon. He knows how urgent it all is. I've heard your father in a temper; it's not very nice …"

"He just kept questioning me. I was frightened." Pala was glad, at least, that she had Cal she could come and talk to if things got desperate.

Chapter 3
FEAR AND ATTACK

At this moment Kim was riding through the crag-like foothills and narrow mountain passes, where he and Plarus had to negotiate rocks and boulders. Here, higher up, it was cooler and less vegetated than down in the valley and going around one bend in the pass he suddenly came to a roadblock. It was the border and several soldiers stood about looking officious. Would they let him through?

As Kim approached the soldiers, he dismounted Plarus and put on as friendly a face as he could. He was nervous; he thought he had seen them lead a horse off around the corner.

"Hullo," he said to the first soldier he came to.

"Let's see that horse of yours." The soldier was abrupt and unfriendly. "We'll take that." The soldier grabbed at the reins but Plarus reared slightly, bucking away.

"No! That's my horse! Don't …! How am I to travel?"

"Where are you headed?" Another soldier had come up to them.

Kim, sweating with fear now, was still trying to hold on to Plarus who was nervous, as more soldiers approached. They had pikes and strutted about self-importantly. Kim walked slowly towards them towing Plarus who, sensing danger, was tugging at the reins.

"I'm on my way to the capital, Trasimid. I obviously can't get there without a horse," Kim said as evenly as he could, with one arm over Plarus's back now to steady the horse as soldiers surrounded them.

"Where have you come from?" the second soldier questioned without answering Kim.

"From Derkia. I'm searching for my uncle."

"And your uncle is in Trasimid?"

"Yes," answered Kim as calmly as he could, though he was now shaking.

"We're taking the horse," the soldier said, pulling the reins forcefully and decisively from Kim. "If you continue on this road, you'll only come upon more soldiers and possibly fighting. They won't be as kind as we are. All we want is the horse and most of the food you've got. We'll leave you a bit of food." This was apparently generous!

The fact was that Kim knew he would not find any food near here. He might as well starve to death, as far as they were concerned.

"Go back the way you came and go left at the first crossroads, there." The second soldier pointed back down the hill from where Kim had come. "The peasants won't hurt you, but we must keep the horse and some food. Give us your bag."

With several soldiers now around him and pikes pointed towards him, the terrified Kim had no choice but to yield up the reins of his beloved Plarus, quickly whispering in his ear: "Be good, my dear Plarus. Make them love you as much as I do. I don't want to leave you, but I think they'll kill me if I don't." And Plarus seemed to understand, nuzzling Kim until the soldiers pulled him away.

With pikes still pointed at him, Kim then handed over his small bag with his food, which the soldiers took, giving him back only bread and tomatoes.

As some of the soldiers were going off with Plarus, one of them called out to him. "Remember! Left at the crossroads!" And, laughing at Kim's alarm, he pointed down the hill.

Kim turned away, hesitating and shaking with anger. His darling Plarus stolen so easily! How would he ever get to Trasimid now?

He ran down the road towards the crossroads and fell onto the grass verge in distress. This was becoming impossible! Had his mother known how difficult it would be? How terrified he would be?

"Come on," he said to himself at last. "I've still got my legs to walk with and my head to think with." And he got up and turned towards the narrow path, which led upwards on the left. My God it was steep! Plarus would not have managed it.

He stumbled up as quickly as he could, wanting to get to the top of the mountain, but it seemed the higher he got – and he must be getting higher by now – the less he could see for scrub and bushes all around him. Unlike most mountain pathways, this path seemed to go almost in a straight line, instead of winding upwards, which would have made a longer path but an easier climb. The higher he got, the more overgrown it became: he was battling not only with the gradient but with thorny scrub that got in the way.

Reaching a little place where he could sit down, he took out the bit of food that the soldiers had left him and started to eat. Once, amidst the noise of the birds, he thought he heard voices, but the sounds went away so he decided he must have been mistaken.

It was colder now and, with not much food in one's belly, a body feels all the colder. As the sun went down, Kim wrapped his warm cover around himself and made a kind of nest amongst some grass. He thought about the gems he had. Should I have bribed the soldiers? he thought. He still had the two gems his mother had given him, which he had carefully hidden on his person: the emerald in his inside back pocket and the amethyst in an inside trouser pocket. He had hidden the diamond in the secret place his mother had taught him about: a little slot on the inside of his waistband, fastened with two threads.

Maybe I should have used the amethyst or the emerald to buy myself out of this terrible situation. Too late! I can't go back there and say, "By the way, I have this gem. Can I have my horse back please?" They would just laugh at me, take the jewel and certainly not give Plarus back.

Also, he remembered they had said that the next lot of soldiers further down that road might have killed him.

No. He was better off climbing this mountain, getting to Trasimid as quickly as he could, however difficult, he decided, as he tried to get some sleep.

Kim slept fitfully, with dreams of being robbed of his blanket and food. He wrapped himself ever tighter into his cover.

As morning dawned with a cloudy mist coming down, Kim ate a few berries, drank the water he still had and plodded on up the mountain. How far was it to the top? He couldn't see ahead in this cloud. In fact, there was nothing to be seen except the occasional small tree, surrounded by bushes, thorns and scrub, which came upon him through the mist.

Suddenly, he heard a loud rush of horses' hooves and shouting. Four horsemen, their faces covered with dirty pieces of cloth and riding strong little mountain horses, were coming at him from the mist above. He stumbled with a thud, back into the bushes nearby, frozen with fear.

"See him?" one shouted. "There he is!" He rushed towards Kim.

"Get him, quick!" another shouted, jumping off his horse.

"Doesn't look as if he's got much …" yet another shouted, leaping adeptly off his own horse.

Kim desperately tried to get up and run back down the mountainside, shouting "I haven't got anything!" But he was surrounded and the bandits' horses knew how to get about this scrub. He wouldn't have a chance. In no time, they had him in a hold.

The third bandit now punched him to the ground as

Kim groaned. Suddenly, another of the bandits rushed up and stabbed him. Kim passed out completely. Two others quickly went through his bag and clothes.

"Nothing!" yelled one of the two searching Kim's pockets. Then: "Here's something!" and he pulled out the emerald.

Kim was now unconscious and bleeding on the ground.

"Come on. Let's get out of here! He's had it anyway ..." another yelled and the four of them got back onto their tough little horses and rode away, down the mountain.

* * *

Kim lay there for some time. Then, coming round, he realised he was not actually dead. He vaguely wondered what they had done to him. He could feel a terrible pain below his left shoulder. Had they stabbed him in the heart? Was he going to die here on the cold mountainside, with no help, freezing to death because he could not move? He started to call out weakly, but not much sound came out and he knew it was useless. There was no-one about. Why waste his energy in calling? But he must move, otherwise he would freeze to death.

Slowly, painstakingly, Kim clambered up the mountain, mainly on his knees, calling as loudly as he could in case there were any peasants or farmers nearby. After what seemed like an age of crawling, he saw a light and pulled himself towards a small cottage. He managed to get to the door and knocked at it as loudly as he could. The next moment a darkness fell over him again.

* * *

At this instant, the door was being opened by the old man who lived there. He immediately pulled Kim into the room as gently as he could, laying him near the fire to warm him.

"Who are you, my fine young man? Very young, I think," he whispered to himself, as he covered Kim with a fur and dragged him near the fire. Seeing the wound, he went to fetch cloths and bandages to clean it. He also brought some of the sauce from the stew he'd had for supper and together with bread tried to feed it to Kim, who kept coming round and swooning again. The old man took hot water from the stove and started to clean the wound gently with the cloths. Then he bound it with the bandages. By now Kim was again unconscious and when the old man felt his forehead, it was burning hot. He put a damp cloth over Kim's head, not daring to take the covers off his body as he had been shivering before, and he went off to gather straw for a bed. This he piled into the corner nearest the fire and then dragged Kim, rolled into a blanket, onto the straw mattress. He gave him as much water as he could, lifting Kim's head and tipping it into his mouth. Then he let Kim sleep.

In the morning Kim was still sleeping as the old man went out to milk the goat and collect any eggs the hens had laid. He brought more logs for the fire and warmed milk up, drinking some of it. Next, he went to Kim and felt his forehead again. Perhaps he just needs water at the moment, the old man thought. He would wait for this young man to awaken to feed him milk. But Kim didn't wake up, he just tossed and turned in a fever all day and all the next night. He awoke briefly the next morning, but still his head was hot. The old man gave him more water and a little milk and Kim fell back to sleep again.

This went on for four days until, on the fifth day, Kim awoke. He watched as the old man put another log on the fire. Then the old man turned around.

"How are you feeling?" he asked Kim, who was now wide awake.

"I'm feeling better … Where am I?"

"You're in my house. My name's Kelin."

"How did I get here?"

"You tell me … I found you collapsed outside my door."

"I was attacked. I was climbing up the mountain path. Some soldiers took my horse so I had to go on foot."

"Soldiers attacked you? Up here?"

"No. They stopped me down in the valley. I'm on my way to Trasimid. But they took my horse and my food and told me it was safer to take the narrow mountain pass. I walked for two days, I think … But then … it must have been bandits who attacked me. They took gold and a jewel from my bag. I think my knife is gone. Only I don't think they found what I had in my … Where are my …"

Kelin pointed towards his bag and clothes folded, near the palliasse.

"Well, I'm glad you managed to keep something from them," Kelin said. "They are vicious. You are lucky not to have been killed."

"I think they thought they had killed me because I passed out. When I came to, I just tried to walk or crawl; then I saw a light... I don't remember much more than that."

"You were collapsed outside the door when I came. And you've had a fever, but it's gone now, I think."

"How long have I been here?"

"Four days."

Kelin went away now to get some broth for him as Kim looked around the one room. When the old man came back, he sat down on the floor next to Kim.

"Here. Drink that. It'll do you good. You haven't had much. Mainly sips of water when you were feverish." He helped him to drink the soup. "I just live here on my own now. My wife died four years ago. There's only me and the goat, a few hens and two donkeys. They grind the corn for me. I manage to live on that, and the bit of land out at the back. The bandits never bother me. There's nothing to take from here. They don't want donkeys. You're lucky, young man … They've killed two travellers up this mountain so far. Traders they were. One was a year ago, down near the road; the other just two months ago, by the stream. They surprised him drinking. Both were knifed, like you."

"I would like to repay you … You've saved my life," Kim said to the old man. "All I've got is a diamond hidden in the top of my trousers, where the robbers didn't look! I was going to give it to my uncle when I find him, so that he can be sure who I am, because I was a child when he last saw me." Kim felt it was necessary to tell this fib to spare the old man from knowing who he really was. "But now I would like you to have the gem."

"Steady on, young man, you're not ready to go off yet. Anyway, what would I do with a priceless gem? No, if you want to repay me, you can get yourself completely healed and strong again and then help me with the roof that has too many holes in it. But only when you're well. It takes time for a wound like that to heal."

"The roof? Yes, I don't think I'm quite up to doing a roof yet." But I need to get on, Kim thought to himself. How am I going to get back in time if I'm here recovering?

"No, I'll do the roof myself," Kelin went on. "You can do other things: fetch water from the stream, find and chop wood, plant and sow seeds, hoeing, seeing to the goat and hens, feeding the donkeys. There's plenty to do."

*   *   *

So Kim started to recover and at the same time he took on gradually more of the chores that needed doing around the cottage, while Kelin started mending the roof.

After four weeks Kelin had fixed the hole in the roof.

"What would I have done without you here, looking after my animals, grinding the corn and planting a new lot in the little meadow?" joked Kelin. "You've been a godsend and I think you are definitely fit now, to go on your journey. I can be sure that there will be no more leaking through my roof when it rains, ruining my books and papers. My buckets can now be put to better use!"

"And I can go over the mountain to Trasimid to look

for Balquin!" said Kim delightedly. He had decided at last to confide in the wise old Kelin about his search – though not about his own origins, for fear of embarrassing the old man.

"When you journey to Trasimid," Kelin said, "you must take one of the donkeys – Modo, I think. Modo's a gentle and kind-hearted donkey with great character. He loves going to the city and seeing the world; ride him always and don't ride any horse on your journey, only a donkey. Not until your task is completed can you ride a horse. Modo will keep you safe from robbers who are not interested in men on donkeys and also – more important – he'll keep you slow. The pace of that animal will lead you to the truth, something we're all searching for; rushing and hurrying can never lead you there because there is no time to think – and we all need time to reflect on things.

"I will give you a package as well as two large sacks of ground maize to take with you. The maize you must sell at the next village, where they're waiting for it at the farm over the mountain. In the spring the bandits go away to spend summer in the lowlands and plains, where they can live outside and get to different places more quickly. I don't think they'll trouble you now. They come back to the mountain caves in the autumn when the weather gets colder again and they huddle together for warmth to discuss their projects.

"With the money for the maize you'll have enough to go on to Trasimid and when you get to the capital, I want you to go and see an old friend of mine, Tiésa. She has a herb shop at the bazaar. Take the package of papers to her and she'll help you to find this man, Balquin. Keep the clothes I have given you because they will help keep you safe. The bandits, if they see you again, are unlikely to recognise you in that old hat. And anyway, they're only interested in signs of wealth. That's part of the reason for the donkey. Tiésa will give you a talisman of great power. This you must guard with your life. If you manage to keep it, the talisman will be sure to see you through the most difficult situations. When you've found Balquin, I want you to meet me in a town called the City of Towers, in the far north of Memarn. I will be there on the seventh of September, every year for the next three years, by the well in the main square."

"It's not going to take me three years!"

"No, but you never know … Listen, if I am not there on the seventh of September, by the central well in the City of Towers, you must wait for three days. I will lead you back over the mountains to avoid the dangerous places. And now, I shall also leave here, because every year before spring I go down to the valley. My daughter lives there with her husband and children and I help them out with the planting and reaping later, in summer."

"What about the goat and the hens? Who'll look after them?"

"They come with me. And then, when I travel on, I can leave them with Murima, my daughter."

"You have been so kind, Kelin. I don't know how to thank you."

"Well, I should thank you. My roof was getting worse

and worse because I never had enough time to get up that ladder – until you came. You can thank me by keeping to the ten things I've told you." Kelin had spent the last evening carefully enumerating ten tasks that Kim had to remember on his journey so as to allow himself to finish his endeavour and to keep safe as well. "Then, we are more likely to meet up in the City of Towers, though anything could happen. It's dangerous, what you are trying to do."

The next day they loaded up the donkeys – Kim's Modo with the two sacks of ground maize and Kelin's donkey with the cart, taking the hens and the goat.

"Thank you for everything, Kelin," said Kim, embracing the old man. "I will do everything you say and see you in the City of Towers."

"Don't forget a word of what I've said. If you forget anything, you'll have a more difficult time. If you keep the talisman safely, you'll be all right in the end." He embraced young Kim fondly, got onto his cart and drove his donkey gently down a nearby, winding track. Kim watched, and before he turned the corner, the old man looked back at Kim, calling, "Farewell, my good prince!"

Kim was dumbstruck! Had he heard correctly? Did Kelin know who he really was? Maybe he had said something in his delirium when he first came to the old man's door. Was that why he knew that Kim's task was difficult and dangerous? Anyway, by the time he recovered from his surprise, the old man was out of sight, hidden by bushes down the track. In a moment he would see him again, further down the path. He waited and when the little cart came into sight, again, Kelin turned once more and Kim waved at him. Then he got onto Modo and, with their heavy load, they ambled slowly up the mountain in the opposite direction, where the land was more open, vegetated with a thin, tough grass.

As Kim moved upwards towards the summit of the little mountain, he tried to memorise what Kelin had said to him.

Number one: sell the maize at the next village on the other side of the mountain, the first farm you come to. Just follow this little path towards the next valley – the track makes a slight right turn towards the village and the farm. It will take three days to get to the farm.

Two: use the money from the maize for the journey onwards and to buy food, apples, et cetera.

Three: at Trasimid find the woman called Tiésa in the marketplace and give her the package of papers.

And, four: she will help you to find Balquin.

Five: keep wearing the old clothes because they will help to make you uninteresting to any robbers.

Six: Tiésa will give you a talisman of great power.

Seven: guard the talisman with your life (that means sew it into the inside of your waistband so that you cannot be robbed of it, he thought).

Eight: after getting the papers and documents off Balquin, go to the City of Towers to meet Kelin. Wait for him there, by the well, on the seventh of September, for three days if necessary.

Nine: Kelin will guide you back on a safe route over

the mountains from the north of Memarn towards Grailand and Strela. The only thing about all this was the time it would take. Kim couldn't afford anything like three years! Even one year, though possible, would be too long in his mind at this moment. He would rather three months! He really had to find Balquin as soon as he could, to get rid of this curse before the *Festival of the King's Reign* at the end of next year, and also to prevent Sagesse being betrothed to some stranger!

Kim went through Kelin's list of the nine key things once more. There was another, tenth thing, but he couldn't for the life of him remember what it was. It was only later, coming down the other side of the mountain that he remembered it.

At that moment he and Modo were still climbing higher and higher and looking at the open blue sky, with its little fluffy clouds, as well as the beautiful view below them. And Kim spent his time memorising the nine things. He knew they were essential to the successful outcome of what he now realised was a dangerous undertaking.

Chapter 4
A BLACK HORSE FOLLOWS

At Koremine Castle, Pala had gone through agonies after realising that, in her anger against her father, she had let out things that she should have kept quiet about. Conversely, King Demble had also realised this. He wouldn't question her any more. She had said enough to make him very nervous indeed.

The day after this, King Demble went to see his general, General Misot, a formidable and cruel man who had so far managed to put down all insurgents and protesters and fill the prisons of Strela.

"All I know, General," said King Demble, "is that he is looking for a stranger who possibly has some secret information; but I don't know exactly where the prince went as he left without my permission and wouldn't tell me where he was going. I want him found before he reaches that stranger and gets hold of that information! It is far too dangerous for him to know these secrets. It could cause unrest and even revolution in the country if it were known. Prince Kim must be found in his search, and stopped at all costs."

"Do you know who he is searching for, Your Majesty?"

asked the general.

"A kitchen boy!" replied the irate king.

"A kitchen boy? You mean there is a kitchen boy who knows state secrets?"

"He *was* a kitchen boy, some twenty years ago. In the castle. Lord knows what he is doing now or where he is. I don't even know his name, though we could possibly get that from one of the servants who have worked in the castle a long time. Cook will probably know him, as she employed him."

"Cook?" repeated the general. "Is that all we have to go on?"

"We didn't bother much at the time. The boy ran away from the castle and we thought he'd drowned. And I think Queen Donata may have known things about him that I never knew. It was the queen, I'm sure, who told the prince about the kitchen boy. You just need to catch up with Prince Kim and see where he goes. It could be Beran, Grailand or even Memarn. If necessary, get rid of the kitchen boy, when you find him. I cannot have this information coming out. It could ruin the royal family!" He stopped for a moment and then added, "But I suppose he's not a kitchen boy, nowadays. It was a long time ago – when my father was on the throne."

"I see. I understand, sir. How many men should I take with me?"

"How many men do you think you'll need? I want them dressed in mufti, ordinary clothes, so they're not recognised. Send them to the places I mentioned and make sure they all know what Prince Kim looks like."

"Yes. Tall – for fifteen, anyway. Good looking, dark hair. I'll only send the ones that know him. About fifty, I should think … We'll find him, sir. He's easy to spot."

Fifty of the army personnel were now sent out to various parts to make inquiries and to search for Prince Kim of Strela. The cook, who had been at the castle from the time of King Strearn, was questioned at length about the boy:

"What was his name?"

"Oh, sir, it was a long time ago. He was only a boy. I think it was something like Bally, or Bolly. I can't remember precisely." But they pressed her and pressed her until she was almost in tears. "Balquin, I think it was. Something like that."

Luckily for Cook, Jovo still worked at the castle, having improved his status to footman. When he was questioned, he knew exactly the name of his old friend: "It was definitely Balquin," Jovo said, when asked. "Why do you want to know?" But no answer was given to his question.

"And do you know why he ran away?" The general fired the next question.

"Not sure, really. We thought he was frightened of something, but I wouldn't know what that was." And after that Jovo and Cook were left in peace.

Meanwhile the king was in a turmoil. What if Prince Kim found this young kitchen boy – who obviously wasn't so young now! How on earth would he do this? How was it that Queen Donata knew so much about it all? And why had he, the king, not questioned his wife properly when she was still alive?

His instinct was to go with the general and his soldiers, but it would not be seemly in a king to be seen searching for his son. He must wait for the general's messengers to tell him when they had found Prince Kim and captured the Balquin person. He was furious; he would just have to sit and wait.

*　*　*

After a night spent at the top of the mountain in a shepherd's hut that Kelin had told him about, Kim and Modo started on their way down over the other side, along the meandering path. When, that afternoon, still high up, they reached a lush little valley, Kim could see that now they only had to follow the fast-flowing mountain stream which became the River Wisees, leading eventually to Trasimid. The air was sweet and warmer than it had been and the birds sang with renewed gusto. Kim caught a fish in the river and cooked it on an open fire. He felt full of hope now and was longing to reach the Memarn capital to meet Kelin's friend and to find Balquin.

The path, widening slightly, had wound round in the grass, through trees, sometimes near the river and sometimes away from it. At one point, as the track approached the river on a bend again, they had moved off it towards the river onto the lovely thick grass, which was so sumptuous here that Modo could gorge himself eating this delicious, green pasture and Kim could eat his fish and watch the water splashing over the little rocks.

Suddenly Kim saw a large, dark animal a bit further on, moving about amongst the trees on this side of the river's bank.

Is that a bear? Kim thought to himself, in some fear, as he didn't know where to hide and he knew that they could climb trees. Oh no, it's a horse, he realised, as it moved through the trees. But where's the rider?

The horse was tall, fine and shiny black, and was grazing near what was now a fast-flowing river. It didn't seem particularly disturbed by Kim, who went to fill his bottle. As Modo continued his munching, the horse went on casually chewing the grass and keeping an eye on them. It had bridle and reins, but was not tethered. As Kim got a full view of the horse, it stopped and looked directly at him for a moment and then carried on chewing.

Kim went back to Modo, tethering him to a tree but giving him plenty of length to move about. He then turned and slowly, carefully moved towards the horse again. "Where on earth is your rider?" he said quietly, as he moved nearer to the horse, looking around to see if there was someone nearby. There was no-one. He went right up to the horse.

"Hullo. What's your name? You seem all alone out here. Who is it who owns such a beautiful creature?"

Kim gently took hold of the reins, stroking the horse's nose. The horse accepted the caress for a moment, but then, as the horse started to back away from him, Kim immediately let go the reins, for fear of frightening it. "Where are you going?" he said as the black horse moved on a few yards. Then it turned to look at him.

"You want me to follow?" So, Kim followed the horse a little way along the bank by the river until he could see a kind of mound. The horse was standing by the mound now, facing him squarely as Kim approached.

When he was nearer, he suddenly realised the mound was a body, all crumpled up, lying on the bank of the river. Looking closely, he saw this was a young man who seemed to have been dead for about a day, knifed in the chest, the same way Kim had been attacked, only the knife had reached this man's heart. So much for Kelin believing that bandits left the mountains at this time of year! This man must have died quickly, Kim thought. He was well dressed and bits of clothing and bags were strewn amongst the tall grass. Kim looked to see if he could find any clue as to who this was, inspecting the clothing, going through all the bags.

After careful searching, he found a large diamond hidden in the dead man's waistband, which the robbers had missed. On one of the man's legs, inside his boot, was an anklet. It was a chain that seemed old and of little value and had an inscription on it: "Aziel". Kim decided to take both the diamond and the anklet to Tiésa and ask her what to do with them. She may be able to find out the identity of the man from the inscription.

With nothing to dig with, Kim managed to bury the man by piling bits of the overhanging bank and clods of grass over him. "I hope I have buried you soon enough …" he muttered as he went back to get Modo.

He left the black horse, because he remembered now what that tenth thing was that Kelin had said to him.

Kelin had specifically warned him against getting a horse, however tempting it might be. In these parts, he said, a horse proclaims you as having money and unless you give it up readily or can fight for it, you will probably be killed for a horse; Kim still mourned the loss of Plarus and wouldn't risk anything like that again. Maybe, he thought, the horse had run away when the robbers had struck, otherwise they surely would have taken it.

Now he and Modo went on their way, along the pathway by the river, down the gentle slopes of this side of the mountain where the grass was plentiful and there were soft hills all around.

Some way further down the road, Kim noticed a kind of echo. He stopped and listened. What could that be? There was no doubt, the clip-clop sound was continuing through the valley; but it did not stop when they stopped. Kim and Modo went on a little more, then stopped again. There it was, the echoing. Now they turned and waited. After a few moments the black horse appeared from round a bend in the road further back. It was following them! What should he do?

"I must not have a horse with me," he thought. But he couldn't help it if a horse insisted on following him. Well, let it. It could follow him to the village; they could have it there.

That night Kim and Modo slept on slopes near to the river, with Modo having gorged himself full of the rich grasses nearby and Kim well satisfied with his afternoon meal of fish that he had caught and cooked. The black horse watched over them from a distance, slightly hidden under a bunch of trees further up the hill.

The next morning at dawn, Kim and Modo continued on their way downhill, with the black horse several hundred metres behind, following like a faithful dog. The horse stayed with Kim and Modo the following night also, at a safe distance, as they camped late and Kim could just make out some lamps in the village. When morning came, they moved on downwards towards the nearest cottages barely visible in the early morning mist.

The first group of cottages proved, on closer inspection, to be the outhouses and farm that Kelin had said would buy both his sacks of maize. They would keep one of them and would later take the other to the market and sell it off. Kim knocked at the door to the main building and a woman came.

"Yes?"

"I've come from Kelin over the mountain. He's asked me to bring these two bags of maize to you."

"Why didn't he come? He usually does a round trip to Trasimid."

"I'm on my way to Trasimid myself. I've business there," Kim said. "So he's sent me instead. He's gone straight to his daughter's in the north. He went with his goat and hens and he's lent me his donkey, Modo. We've had a good ride over the mountain."

She knew he must be telling the truth, because how would a stranger know Kelin had a daughter in the north? The woman was just about to ask him in, when she saw the horse standing a good hundred metres away on the track.

"Whose horse is that?"

"That horse has been following me down the mountainside. It led me to its owner, who must have been killed by bandits. I buried the man but left the horse and now he's followed us down." And Kim told the woman about finding the horse and the dead man. But he left out telling her about the diamond and the anklet because, he thought, it would be enough for the villagers to have the black horse. "But, you see," Kim went on, "I don't need a horse because I have the wonderful Modo, Kelin's donkey!"

Actually, he would have really relished a beautiful black horse to go galloping through the countryside and to reach his destination in extra-quick time. But things never happen exactly the way you want them to, so despite his wish for the horse, he said he was happy with Modo, the modest little donkey.

"We can buy the maize off you and give you a very good price for it if the horse goes with it," the woman said, eyeing the horse carefully and seeing it was a good one. "Just a moment," she said, and went back into the house. A moment later she was out again with a bowl in her hands. "Take these oats to get him to come into our farm."

Kim did as she said, went over to the horse and fed the oats to him while leading him firmly into the farm and giving the reins into the hands of the woman, who was more than delighted with her bargain.

Then Kim went on his way, minus two bags of maize and a horse, and loaded up with a fair amount of money in his pocket.

Here in the wider valley, the path opened out even more; it was still high up, but Modo, delighted now to have got rid of the heavy maize bags, fairly spun downwards. And Kim was almost as eager as Modo to see what their destination would bring, but anxious also that he had so much to do: find a man who may have been hiding for about twenty years; try to get from this man a secret that he had spent the same amount of time keeping hidden; and then keeping himself incognito, with the help of Kelin's old hat, to make sure he was not recognised as a prince.

"Look at the view, Modo!" Kim said in wonder, as they came round a bend, looking down onto Trasimid, the great capital of Memarn, below them in the valley.

Chapter 5
TIÉSA AND THE BLACKSMITH

Trasimid was a beautiful, old, walled city with lookout posts all along its ramparts and north, south, east and west arches as entry gates into the city.

Kim and Modo entered through the arch at the western gate. Here the narrow street was busy with people and flanked on either side with closely packed houses and shops with colourful awnings. The noise, the talking and shouting, the clatter of horses, donkeys and carts on the cobbled streets, the smell of the crowds, of cooking foods, the perfumes all filled Kim and Modo with a sense of excitement, compared with the peace and calm of the countryside.

"Which way to the bazaar?" Kim asked a nearby seller of cooked meats.

"The bazaar? Why that's at the very centre of the city." And the man described in detail where it was.

"Thank you," Kim said to the man and he and Modo moved on towards the centre.

On reaching the bazaar, it was so crowded that Kim dismounted and walked along the narrow streets, towing Modo, who was delighted with the sweets and cakes on show. Soon, they came to a mass of covered passages with little shops, their wares spilling out onto stands for Modo to nibble at, if he had the chance.

"Do you know of a herbalist near here?" Kim asked another stallholder.

"You'll find a herbal shop about three minutes away. First you take a left turning and then immediately right, and you can't miss it," the man said. "It's a bit of a maze." And Kim wondered whether he would ever find his way out again. But that's the kind of feeling a new place gives you, when you don't know your way around. In time Kim would know all the side-alleys and all the friendly faces in this buzzing bazaar. At the moment it was taking all his energy to keep one eye out for the herbal shop, another for beggars and a third checking Modo's overwhelming desire for sweetmeats and flowers, both of which were in abundance here.

Someone, perhaps Trent, had told him that Balquin could have become a beggar. So Kim now inspected the beggars he passed as Modo took the chance to seriously scrutinise the delicious things on the stalls or, at one point, have a discreet munch on a woman's flowers sticking out of her shopping basket.

But Kim didn't talk to any of the beggars; he knew he must follow Kelin's instructions and find Tiésa first. On the other hand, he couldn't help looking at the poverty-stricken beggars and wondering. Some of them looked ill or handicapped; Kim suddenly had a terrible sense of fear. What if Balquin were dead? Who would have the information he needed?

Kim reached the little shop, overflowing with herbs of every kind, with a shelf at the back covered with jars of spices and medicines. Inside, were yet more spices of all colours, bottles filled with liquids and tinctures and glass jars with powders of varying hues. There was an older woman sitting inside the glass area, talking animatedly to a young woman about her child's illness. She had kind, laughing eyes with her white hair tied under a little cap in a knot at the back of her head. She got up, selected three jars off the shelves, tipped a little powder from each into a paper pouch, closed it, shook it for a few seconds, then gave it to the woman. She then went outside and picked a few sprigs of dried thyme from the stall, wrapping that into a pouch also. The young woman gave her a few coins, thanked her warmly and left.

Meanwhile, Kim had tied Modo to a nearby post away from temptation and had taken out of his bag the packet that Kelin had given him. He had been watching through the glass as the older woman had spoken to the young woman. Inside, there was barely room for one person and, at the back, a screen and curtain which perhaps hid another room. Eventually, when the old woman came out, Kim went to her.

"Are you Tiésa?" he asked.

"I certainly am!" said the herbalist.

Kim bowed slightly to her and presented her with the package.

"This is from my good friend Kelin in the Binon Mountains, near the River Wisees. He sends you his warmest greetings and says you might possibly be able to help me in my search."

Tiésa asked him to sit down and then untied the string on the packet. Inside was a wad of loose papers filled with close writing. She looked at them for a moment and then put them carefully back into the paper, tying the string around the packet again. She then put the packet of papers into an inside pocket of her overall and turned, looking straight at Kim: "And what is your name …?"

"My name is Kim." He had no fear; it was a common enough name.

"Ah. I see," said Tiésa. "Wait here, would you, a moment?" With that she disappeared behind the curtain into another part of the shop; little or large, Kim had no idea. A moment later she was back.

"Will you please take this? I think you know its value and what to do with it."

"Thank you. Kelin has told me exactly what to do." Kim looked at what had been placed in his hands. It was a palm-sized stone carving of a woman's head. He felt a tinge of recognition but could not place it.

Tiésa was speaking to him again. "You must guard this with your life. Look at it now and remember it. Then you must hide it. But first, have you somewhere to stay?"

"Well, I've just arrived and haven't really had time …"

"A friend of mine," Tiésa interrupted, "has a nice little place near the north gate. Sabio is his name and if you tell him I have sent you he will give you a room and a place for your donkey. I can come there in a couple of hours and we will go for some supper, if you'd like."

"That's very kind of you," said Kim. And Tiésa proceeded to explain precisely how to get to Sabio's house from the bazaar.

Out in the warm May sun again, he towed Modo back through the market in the direction that Tiesa had told him. They were at last in the city of Trasimid and Kim could not believe how far he had come, as they went along one of the main roads, taking in the animation of the city, with its busy traffic of people riding and rushing about on foot, talking, shouting, bargaining and generally carrying on.

As Kim watched some dapper-looking riders on horseback coming towards him down the main road, he suddenly recognised the face of the rider nearest him. Had he not seen this young man before? Quickly, instinctively, Kim pulled Kelin's old hat down, low over his face, so he could just make out what was happening in front of him. He now moved quickly into a narrow side street, with Modo as cover. Thank God for Kelin's old hat and clothes! Kim stood, half-hidden in a great double-doorway of the side street, watching the five or six men on horseback as they stopped to consult together. He could see Laurent with them, another of his father's army, whom he had talked to on several occasions and who had once shown him how to brush down a horse to make it sleek and shiny. And thank God Kim was with Modo, the donkey! Had any of them seen him? It didn't seem so. They were not looking down this side street.

Kim's heart was pounding nineteen to the dozen and he was sweating. He tried the handle of the door and, with a slight creak, half of the great double door opened wide. Kim pulled Modo into the vast stone hallway which led onto a garden-like courtyard through to the back. Inside, it was dark and cool compared to the bright warmth outside in the street. He was safe, at least for the moment. But Kim knew there could only be one reason his father's men were in Trasimid. They were here because of him. Somehow, King Demble had got wind of his purpose here – proof that something important must have happened that night of the quarrel, otherwise the king would not have sent these men so far. But what had really happened?

He tied Modo to one of the rings fixed in the wall in the large, dark, open vestibule and he squatted down, his breathing getting lighter and easier moment by moment. All these men – six of them he had counted – after him? How would he be able to search for Balquin? Should he hand himself over to the men? Give up the search? Return home to Pala and Sagesse empty handed? Of course, Kim didn't know that his father had married the greedy, frivolous Drina, and that she was now in the process of making sure all the riches he had amassed went nowhere else but into her own, grasping little hands. No. To go back now wasn't an option. He must keep going, whatever. He would just have to be extra careful: keep on wearing Kelin's old clothes; possibly talk to Tiésa about his predicament; tell her the full story as he had been ashamed to tell Kelin, who himself had probably guessed some of it. He must stay looking like a peasant, as he did at the moment. The guards would not be searching for anyone wearing old clothes!

Reassured in his own mind that he could outwit them, Kim sat in the great, empty hallway for a good hour to make sure they would all be well and truly gone. When, at last, he cautiously ventured outside, he looked around to try and see any further sign of them, edging towards the nearby main road again and, seeing none of them, he went back for Modo.

After another quarter of an hour along the route that Tiésa had described, he and Modo reached a dusty road, lined with low, well-spaced, modest houses, each with their own courtyard in front. They went into one of the courtyards. The house at the far end of it was built with a series of rooms that came out on both sides, like arms, around the courtyard, with pillars supporting a curved veranda all around. At the centre of the courtyard, seated by a little well, an old man sat carving some wood.

"Have you got a room, by any chance, sir?" Kim asked him. "Tiésa, the herbalist, said you might have a spare room."

"Tiésa?" The old man smiled and made a gesture for him to sit at the well, then moved slowly towards the back of the courtyard near the house.

"Bava!" he called loudly. "Bava!" There was the sound of running footsteps and a young woman appeared. The father and daughter conferred quietly and then Bava came forward.

"Just for you?" she asked.

"Yes. And somewhere for the donkey," Kim answered smiling. "My name is Kim."

"Well, you can sleep here." She was moving now

towards the courtyard entrance, opening a door to the side, under the veranda. "The donkey can stay outside." Bava indicated a ring in one of the pillars holding up the low roof running around the edge of the courtyard; there were two troughs nearby, one of water the other of hay. Kim tied Modo up and Bava then led him into the room, which was small and dark but cool because of the thick walls.

"Thank you." said Kim. "How much is it?"

"Twenty crowns for a month."

Kim gave Bava the money, put down his bag and followed her out into the courtyard. He suddenly realised that he was still clutching tightly in his hand the talisman that Tiésa had given him at the bazaar. He had been holding it all this time. Perhaps it really was lucky and had protected him from being seen by his father's soldiers!

As Kim and Bava came back into the courtyard, Tiésa was entering it from the road.

"I had a rather frightening adventure on the way here which delayed me." He looked over at Bava. "I should have been here sooner …"

"Oh. I see," said Bava. "Well, you managed to get here, so that's all right! There are soap and towels in the room and if you want something to eat, I can bring you something."

"We are off to the gardens for some supper," said Tiésa. "And I want to hear all about your adventure!"

*   *   *

Half an hour later he was seated with Tiésa in a beautiful, hillside garden with little lemon trees and high-up vines draped around in terraces overlooking Trasimid. People here were eating various dishes of food: fish, meats and colourful vegetables filled the tables. Kim and Tiésa had chosen a higher table and were being served fish dishes with rice and nuts and spicy vegetables.

"And all you know about this man, Balquin, is that he was a servant and he overheard your family quarrel …?" Tiésa asked.

"And he left just after Queen Porla, my grandmother, died. Apparently, he fled in fear of his life."

Because of Kelin's last call to him: "Farewell, my prince!" Kim had decided to tell Tiésa everything about his background. In fact, being now sure his father had sent men out to search for him, he told Tiésa about what had happened today.

"So, you're a prince, are you?" Tiésa said after a while of silent thought. "Kelin's done a good job of disguising you!" She laughed at him warmly.

But Kim didn't feel like laughing. "It's not nice being hunted down …"

"I don't think you're actually being hunted down. I mean, they're not out to kill you, are they?"

"No, I suppose not if my father sent them. But I'm sure it's something to do with my search. It must be serious if he's prepared to send men all this way. I wonder how he knows what I am trying to do."

"Are you sure they were looking for you?"

"I wasn't prepared to ask them that!" Kim laughed.

"Well, disguised or not, *I* am going to treat you as an ordinary person. And, from what you've said, it's only *thought* that Balquin left in fear of his life. We don't know that for sure, although it sounds possible," Tiésa went on. "And then, you say, he went to Derkia and stayed in the tavern you worked at."

"If it was him. Apparently, he worked there for a month and then went off to Memarn and some years later was seen by someone who said he was a blacksmith or a cartwright in Trasimid. It was all a long time ago. He may even have died."

"Or he may not be a blacksmith or cartwright any more," said Tiésa. "Balquin is an unusual name. It should be straightforward finding him. I'll make some enquiries and report back to you in three days. We can meet here and I'll tell you what I've found out. He may still be frightened about what happened, even though it was so long ago!"

"Frightened?" asked Kim.

"Yes … well, you said he ran away in fear of his life. Whatever it was he heard must have frightened him a lot."

"I suppose so."

"And why did your mother make you promise to find him?"

"When she was dying, she said the curse of this had affected the family and the whole country and would go on unless it was broken. She said that my children and each following generation had to be protected from it."

"And what is the curse? How does this curse show itself?"

"It's difficult to explain. I have quarrels with my father all the time; my sister is tearful and silent; there is great poverty and want, as well as illness in Strela, even for people who work hard. I've seen it myself; they have little to eat. But my father doesn't care and lets corruption, crime and banditry take over. My mother said the danger with a curse is it makes children become like their fathers, whether they are bad or not." Kim now looked anguished. "I really don't want to become like my father. She said I must find a way not to be afraid and I think you can only do that by being yourself and doing difficult things."

"I think that is right," said Tiésa.

"The thing is, Father's corrupt ministers look after themselves rather than the people whose lives they are responsible for. She said the people chosen by my father to get rid of crimes and misery tell lies and pretend everything's all right, when it's obvious things are not all right. They make sure their own nests are well feathered; they strut about and smirk, but care little for the people they should look after. I've seen it!" he exclaimed. "The people become slaves to the land, but remain hungry themselves!

"In Beran, north of Strela, King Ambab gets rid of the bad ministers. He makes sure his countrymen and women are well and safe; he makes sure his ministers are honest and where he finds they are not, he dismisses them. People are contented there. That is the curse on my country that I've got to remove.

"In Strela, my father's ministers follow his selfish

ways, which gives him the sense that he is powerful."
Kim looked pleadingly at Tiésa. Would she understand?
Finally, he said: "my mother was sure the key was that
terrible quarrel that only Balquin heard. That's why I
have to find him."

"Did she say anything else?"

"Well … she said that although she was not born into
the family, she had experienced this curse in the same
way as Queen Porla. She said people get sucked into the
evils and forget about their real desires and hopes. They
become happy to live in a selfish way that does harm
to others and they become insensitive to their own pain
and the pain they inflict. But if one person takes courage,
others start to take courage and follow. That's what she
whispered to me as she was dying."

Tiésa sat in thought for a moment. Eventually she
asked, "And did you say all this to Kelin?"

"No," Kim replied with care. "No I didn't, because at
that time I was frightened, and when I reached Kelin's I
was so ill that I didn't want anyone to know who I was.
But I think Kelin knew, anyway."

"Kelin is a wise man," said Tiésa. "Nothing much
gets past him!"

"Perhaps I said things in my delirium without
realising."

"Or it's possible he just knew. At any rate, what I have
given you …" here the old woman gave a long look at
Kim, "that will protect you as long as you keep it."

Kim nodded seriously and Tiésa murmured, "I
wonder what gave you the courage to tell me all this …"

"I think it was the horse," Kim said. "Kelin said I should not ride a horse until I knew my search was completed and my task accomplished. But the black horse I saw really wanted me to ride it. I didn't, though." Kim then proceeded to tell Tiésa about the beautiful black horse and the dead man he had buried.

"That's probably the reason!" The old woman smiled. "You resisted the temptation to take it and ride it. You did something quite difficult, for you. And that gave you confidence and you continued your way on Kelin's Modo – which means you arrived here!" They both laughed.

"There is something I forgot to give you, regarding that," said Kim, and he undid the loop he had made in his waistband. "I know we must try to find Balquin … but the dead man had an anklet …" He pulled out the anklet and gave it to Tiésa. "And this …" He then put the large diamond into Tiésa's hand. "Would you be able to keep them safe for me?"

Tiésa looked surprised, inspecting first the diamond, then the anklet.

"'Aziel'," she said, reading the name on the plate side of the little chain. "Obviously the name of the dead man. He was a young man, you say, but this is an old anklet, very old. But not very valuable, I think. I will certainly make inquiries about the man. As to this," she held up the diamond, "I don't mind looking after it for you. But if we can't return it to the dead man's family, I think Kelin should have it. You can take it to him when you meet him in the City of Towers. And now I must go," she added, taking both the diamond and the anklet. "I will see you here in three days. You must make inquiries of your own about this man and we'll see what we both have then. You know your way back, don't you?" Kim nodded his assent and with that the lively old woman was off, waving to Kim as she left the garden.

Kim sat there for a while longer, watching the people eat and talk, and taking in the sounds and smells of the city. He liked Tiésa; she was easy-going and humorous. He knew he would have to fight his own battles, but decided he had an ally here, in Kelin's friend. A weight had been lifted, though he still had it all to do, and quickly.

* * *

He awoke early the next morning, gave Modo hay and water, and drank the tea with dates and sweetmeats that Bava had brought for him, taking one to Modo for a treat. Under Bava's directions he then started off on foot to the other side of town, to search for blacksmiths, having made sure of the big, old hat that Kelin had given him and a slightly ragged look about his clothes so that he wouldn't be easily recognised. Bava had told him that the way to the blacksmiths' side of town would not take him on main roads at all, so he was fairly easy in his mind.

He felt hopeful and excited as he walked along the outskirts of the city, with its sparse houses and the few gardens beyond the outer wall.

If Balquin is still alive and working as a blacksmith, Kim thought, he will surely be glad to give up such a hard life for one of comfort. I will be able to take him back to Strela and make him rich. No-one will need to know who he, Balquin, is or once was. As soon as the secret has been told to me, Balquin will have nothing more to fear. I will never tell a soul. Kim liked the idea of the generosity he would bestow on the poor but worthy Balquin, when he found him. At last, he thought, poor Balquin will feel safe enough to return to his homeland, which he must have longed to do all these years.

When he reached the part of town where the many workshops and smithies were, Kim was almost smiling with pleasure at the thought of what he would do when he found Balquin.

He went into the first blacksmith's he came to.

Inside, the blacksmith was hammering at a forge. A horse stood tethered nearby, waiting to have his new shoes fitted.

"You come for a shoeing?" the blacksmith asked Kim, stopping for a moment in the heat of the forge.

"I'm looking for someone and I wondered if you could help me."

"Who's that then?" asked the blacksmith, starting to hammer again.

"It's a long time ago," said Kim. The blacksmith stopped hammering. "A man who was said to have become a blacksmith or a cartwright, named Balquin. I need his assistance on an important matter …"

"Balquin? Never heard of him. No, don't know …

Sorry. Why don't you try Jolin, the cartwright?"

"Where is he?"

"Only five minutes up along this road."

So, Kim set off again along the road. The sun was getting hot now and he was glad of the shade of the trees which lined this road.

At the cartwright's the man he thought must be Jolin was sitting inside turning spokes on a lathe for a wheel. Kim asked again, "Have you any knowledge of an old friend of my family, Balquin, from Grailand, who I believe became a cartwright or a blacksmith about twenty-five years ago?"

"Twenty-five years ago. That's a while," the cartwright said. "I know most of them around here. Are you sure he's still in the city?"

"He was seen here, working either as a cartwright or blacksmith." Kim's confidence was ebbing away fast. "Striking-looking man, apparently."

"Balquin, Balquin … No. I can't say I've ever … Well, there was one, a man who came from abroad. A long time ago, that was. Could have been Balquin. He was supposed to be pretty good. A blacksmith he was, not a cartwright. You could ask Old Plosit, up the road," he said, pointing. "Just a bit further up the hill, the third workshop along. You can't miss it. He's the oldest one around here. Knows everyone."

Kim thanked Jolin and moved quickly on, up the road. When he arrived at Plosit's smithy, he was hot and thirsty.

"Are you Plosit?" Kim asked as boldly as he could.

"I am. What can I do for you?" The old man watched Kim for a moment, seeing his hot, perspiring face on this warm spring day. "Would you like a glass of tea?"

"I would, please. If you can spare it …"

Old Plosit got up, poured tea from an urn into a glass and gave it to Kim.

"Thank you," Kim murmured, taking a sip. "I've been sent by Jolin the cartwright, who said you may be able to help me."

"What do you want help with then, young man?"

"My name is Kim, sir, and I am trying to find an old friend of my father's who became a cartwright or a blacksmith, I'm not sure which, and is named Balquin. Do you know of him? It was a long time ago."

"Balquin …? Yes. I remember him. A wild young man. Very nervy and difficult, but a wonderful worker. He worked for me for a while. That was more than twenty years ago I should think. Very bright he was, but fairly crazy."

"In what way crazy?" asked Kim.

"I think he'd had some terrible experience."

"Do you know what that was?"

"Been at the heart of some political intrigue, something, I don't know. He was difficult, I remember that. Left after about six months."

"And do you know where he is now?"

"Not really, no. I heard he changed his name, left the city or something. Good at his trade though, as a blacksmith. Very good." Plosit turned away from Kim, back to his forge and hammer. He repeated, murmuring aloud to himself, "Good at it, though." Then, turning back to Kim, Plosit said, "He could hammer out a horse's shoe in no time at all. Gifted, I would call it."

"Is he still a blacksmith?" Kim persisted, as Old Plosit turned his back on him again. "Would he be working in the same trade?" Kim was bewitched with Plosit's talk of the man who held all his secrets. *Gifted*, he had said.

"How would I know? If he had any sense, he would be. A good trade, this. Keeps you busy and with a reasonable living!"

Kim looked at the old, tumbledown workshop where Plosit had been working for at least twenty years. He marvelled that this man could be so happy with his modest living, while others wealthier than he was complained of not having enough.

Plosit now seemed to have completely lost interest in his young questioner and was back hammering away. Yet Kim needed to know more.

"What makes you think he changed his name?" he went on loudly, moving towards the back of the shed, trying to get Plosit's attention through the noise. "Have you heard what his new name is?"

"Look, young man," Plosit looked annoyed now. "I don't know. Right? I can't remember how or why I think he changed his name. Maybe it'll come to me, as things sometimes do. Maybe it won't. Now, I've got work to do here!"

"And you've no idea where he went?"

"No idea whatever! He just disappeared one day. That's it. Now get going before I chase you out with these!" And he lifted out of his fire some red-hot tongs, which had Kim backing away and out of the forge.

If only dear, irate Old Plosit could remember! This was so important. But maybe he never really knew. Kim couldn't tell. It was just too tantalising to be so close to this man who had actually worked with Balquin and yet to have practically no more information than that Balquin was a good – nay *gifted* – blacksmith and that he might have changed his name.

"Thank you!" Kim shouted into the forge, hoping that Plosit would hear. He wanted to remain on the good side of Plosit; despite the blacksmith's vagueness, Kim might need him again. Perhaps when he was in a better mood.

Kim now made his way slowly, dejectedly back to the other side of town. How was he to find Balquin if he had changed his name? It was becoming an impossible task.

Chapter 6
SPILLED TOMATOES

When he got back to his room, he ate some olives and cheese, which he got from Bava, and while he was wondering what to do next he fell asleep on the divan.

An hour and a half later, Kim awoke in a sweat. He had dreamt he had come across a child who was dying. He had picked him up to try to find him a doctor, but then his father, King Demble, came and started to laugh and joke. And each time Kim turned to take the child away, his father stood in front of him, preventing him from moving. In the end King Demble was holding on to Kim to stop him from moving away and Kim was terrified his father would discover the talisman hidden in his waistband and he was shouting, "Let me go! Let me go!" Then he woke up.

He washed his face in an effort to get rid of the nasty feeling the dream had left him with and eventually sat down on the divan to try and think of something else. All he could think was that he didn't know where to turn. Of course, he still had the meeting with Tiésa in a couple of days, and Tiésa did say she would make inquiries herself. He wondered whether he should tell her that Balquin might have changed his name. But he didn't want to bother her as she was obviously busy with her work. It was surely going to be difficult for Tiésa to spend time on Kim's problem. True, Kelin had said that Tiésa would help to find Balquin, but he felt reluctant to presume further on the kind herb doctor's generosity.

Suddenly he realised that of course he could go back to Old Plosit and ask him who else might be able to help him find Balquin. After all, Balquin might have had friends or other connections and Plosit might possibly know them. Kim had been too desperate to think of asking when he was there.

Giving Modo more hay and water on the way out and waving to the old man who was, as usual, sitting by the well, carving his wood, Kim went off again towards the other side of town.

It was cool now and he walked fast. He came to a wide road on the crest of a hill, where some stalls were selling fruit nearby. He looked at the fruit and vegetables piled decoratively up on the stalls. Just in front of him a woman was buying tomatoes. He watched as they were piled into several bags and the woman took the bulging bags in her arms, trying at the same time to put her purse away into her bag. But suddenly, the woman unaccountably stepped back, bumping into Kim as he tried to get out of her way, lurching backwards into him with her tomatoes falling all about.

"Oh, oh! What have you done!" she cried out loudly.

At the same moment three boys ran up, grabbed her

purse, which she was still holding in her hand, and ran off with it.

Kim, seeing all this flash in front of him, shouted and turned to run after the three boys, yelling at the top of his voice, "Thieves! Get back here!"

But they disappeared quickly, into the maze of streets nearby, before he even had a chance to see where they had gone. He searched around the narrow side roads and alleys for a while, but he had lost them completely. As he returned to the wide road with the market stalls, a crowd had gathered around the woman and her spilled tomatoes. She was still shouting and wailing loudly. At the sight of Kim coming back towards her she started up again, giving a great yell, pointing at him, shouting towards him: "There he is! There's the boy!"

People from the crowd now converged threateningly on Kim, as he moved towards them. But Kim, not understanding the situation, called over to the woman as he approached.

"I couldn't find them! They disappeared!"

"He was in on it!" shouted the woman to the growing crowd. "He was the one who made me spill my tomatoes. And then he helped them escape with my purse!"

By now Kim was being held tightly by a few men in the crowd and was struggling to get out of their grip.

"No! No … you bumped into me and spilled your tomatoes!"

"He's lying!" the woman screamed, as she rushed around the men who had Kim in their grasp.

"That's not true …" Kim shouted. "I tried to catch

the thieves. I ran after them when they took your purse, but I couldn't find them. It really wasn't me!" But Kim's desperate words were ignored.

There are always some people who have to blame others when something goes wrong in their lives. It counted for nothing that Kim had actually been trying to help the woman.

"He took it from me! I saw!" she insisted again. Nothing would change her certainty that Kim was to blame for the theft of her purse. A law-officer was called to the scene and he searched Kim thoroughly.

"I can't find the purse," he said. Then, delving into another of Kim's pockets, he exclaimed, "But wait a moment! What is this?" And he pulled out Kelin's maize money, which Kim had stupidly forgotten to give to Sabio or Bava for safekeeping. "So much money on a poor boy like you?"

"I have just been paid by a farmer for some maize. That's my money."

The law-officer turned to the hysterical woman. "How much money was in your purse?"

"Oh no, sir. It wasn't as much as that …" The woman looked overwhelmed at the amount the officer had found on Kim.

"But I've only got that because I was paid for something. It's not mine – it belongs to my friend." Again, his protest went unheard in the general excitement and hubbub of people around, who thought they had caught a thief.

Kim had stopped struggling by now. He was simply

exhausted, trying to make them understand how completely innocent he was. He felt sickened that his behaviour had been so misunderstood; sickened with fear, as the law-officer decided to take him over to the law office, threatening him not only with prison but with execution if he was found guilty.

Once at the law office, a tall, grey-brick building not far from the little market, he was again briefly searched. All his belongings, other than his clothes, were taken from him, as he continued to protest:

"But I am innocent! I was trying to help her after she crashed into me!"

"She says the opposite," said the sullen, bored officer, who had taken over from the first officer; he had been given all the so-called details of this case and also had searched Kim, finding only Kelin's money in his pocket. Luckily, they didn't imagine they should look for any gems this poor-looking boy had on him.

"Can I please send a message to the people I'm staying with?" Kim asked as politely as he could, though he was sick to his stomach inside.

"Probably glad to be rid of you, aren't they? A thief like you?" The law-officer laughed snidely.

"I'm not a thief, and they are expecting to see me. I have to tell them what's happened!"

"Ah, these important people!" said the law-officer sourly. But all the same he came over to the bars of the cell with a note pad. "Right; who are they? We'll see if we can get a message over to at least one of them!"

With a trembling hand, Kim then wrote onto the

paper the names and addresses of both Tiésa and Sabio and the law-officer ambled back to his desk. Flinging the notebook down onto it, he then proceeded to ignore Kim completely.

How had he got into this mess? How could it happen that a person trying to be helpful could land up accused and liable not only to be sent to prison, but to be executed? What kind of a country was this? And did this kind of thing go on in other countries? What about Strela? Kim's mind was racing too fast and his sense of fury at his situation was making him tremble. Fear made him almost tearful and, during a sleepless night, one or two tears did fall onto the pillow-less, hard mat of a bed.

* * *

After three days no-one had been to see Kim and he was now desperately anxious about Tiésa. What must she be thinking? What must Sabio and Bava be thinking? Where did they imagine he had got to?

"I'm sorry it took me so long to find you!" It was Tiésa, on the fourth day. "I've been racking my brains as to where you could be. And here you are! Why on earth ...?" Poor Tiésa looked as if she'd had a few sleepless nights herself. Kim told her the story and she was aghast at the ignorant cruelty of the people.

"Since then, they've just kept me under lock and key. They've threatened execution if I'm found guilty; they haven't offered me a lawyer or told me when I'm to be tried. It's more or less the woman's word against mine.

And the whole town – or rather the marketplace – now think they saw me run off with the thieves."

"Well," Tiésa said, looking seriously at Kim, "I'm glad to see you're still wearing the same old clothes!"

"Oh, these rags!" Kim managed a laugh. "It's partly my ragged condition that makes me look guilty, with all the money I had on me."

"I'll find out when you're going to be tried and come to court as a character witness. I'm a respected citizen. They'll believe me if I say you were sent by my friend to sell the maize and that's where you got the money."

"But will they believe that I was actually trying to catch the thieves?"

"I don't know. You can never know what will happen ..." Despair tinged her voice. The following day, Kim was taken to the court of law. The judge sat on his bench and looked coldly at young Kim.

"Another ruffian, is he?" he said loudly to the clerk at law, sitting next to him. Kim opened his mouth to protest but his defending lawyer stopped him, whispering: "The chances of you being able to get off this charge are small, despite the fact that it's obvious you are a newcomer to our city."

"How could I know those thieves?" Kim whispered back. "I had only arrived in the city a couple of days before!".

"Yes. But these people think robbers have a fraternity all over the different lands; that they all know each other and help each other. We have a terrible problem with brigands who move around the country robbing and killing."

"Yes …" said Kim, thinking of the attack on him and the dead man by the river. "I know that to my cost."

* * *

The trial lasted a day. The woman, who was called Gilina, swore blind that Kim had knocked into her so hard that all her tomatoes had fallen about and she was confused. Then the robbers had snatched her purse and she saw Kim running off with them.

When Tiésa got to the witness stand she testified that Kim was a newcomer to the city and had been sent by her friend who had provided him with a donkey and maize to sell and was preparing to meet him on the north border.

"But why," asked the prosecutor, "would someone do that – give him a donkey to ride and maize to sell? For what reason?"

"He is to collect something from me," replied Tiésa, "for my friend."

"And what is that?" the prosecutor demanded.

"It is a special herb which is a cure for a disease that his daughter has. He himself couldn't come because he has to help his daughter and son-in-law with all the work on the farm, so he sent Kim instead."

"What is the name of the herb?" the prosecutor asked.

"It's called *thuja*," Tiésa answered calmly.

This seemed to somewhat satisfy the judge and he summed up by saying: "It is fairly clear that Kim had no hand in the robbery and I believe him when he says he was trying to catch the robbers. If he *had* caught them", the judge said, "it might have been a different story. But as he did *not* catch the robbers, Kim will have to serve a minimum of one month in Trasimid jail for being so careless as to lurch into Gilina. This," the judge said, "caused the tomatoes to spill and thus we had a situation where the robbers were able to take her purse." He turned to Kim. "After your time in prison, your money will be returned, minus a fine of two-hundred crowns," the judge concluded.

Now, one month in prison compared to say, one year, may not sound long, but when all you have done is actually try to come to someone's assistance and that person turns on you, then the whole thing seems too much. The only thing that gave Kim any comfort at this moment was that Modo was being well taken care of by Bava and Sabio and that he would be allowed to keep his own clothes – though, he complained to Tiésa, "The talisman didn't help me much this time, did it?"

"It's not always possible to know whether it helped. They could have found you guilty and condemned you to death. So, I think it has helped, Kim, just as it helped you get away when you saw your father's men." He was forced to admit to Tiésa that things could have been much worse.

*   *   *

Kim was eventually deposited into a large prison cell, with about fifty prisoners of different ages and descriptions. This was a rough, raucous and unfriendly place and, although all the men here were suffering similar circumstances, they strangely seemed to have no sympathy for one another. They were mainly much older and all talking full blast with one another, terrifying Kim with their loudness; he decided not to engage with them and kept to himself.

When food was brought, it was practically inedible: dry bread and a watery "soup", which tasted of nothing much and if you were lucky had a pea or a small bit of over-boiled meat floating about in it. In the morning, breakfast was a thin gruel which made Kim retch as soon as he looked at it.

Kim sat in his corner in silence.

The loud ones are used to being here and don't care, he thought, listening and watching. It's the silent ones who, like me, are perhaps wrongly imprisoned. I am in here, wasting time, doing nothing when I should be searching for Balquin! His mind went to Sagesse. What would she think of me if she could see me now? he thought. What is she doing now? Who is she seeing? Who is she with? Does she know of my feelings for her? Does she know I want her to wait for me? Will her mother betroth her to someone else? Why didn't I tell her more about my journey? I didn't because I couldn't. I had no idea it would lead me into prison. What would she do if she knew that my father's men were looking for me? Does she know how sad my mother was before she died? Does she know how unhappy I am?

All these thoughts and questions flew at Kim, making

him feel both dejected and bombarded with affliction, particularly at night, when lights were left on and the noise of dreams, nightmares and arguments persisted.

One night, as usual trying to block his ears to get some sleep, he heard a man sobbing quite near to him. The man on the mattress next to his was weeping quietly, as if he were trying to suppress the sounds but could not prevent his distress.

Kim lay there, listening to the sobbing for a while, then he turned towards the man who was in such anguish.

"What is it, friend?" Kim asked him. "Talk to me about it, you may as well. While you're sobbing like that I'll never be able to get any sleep ..."

But the man did not answer him and continued to sob. In the end Kim blocked his ears and managed to get a few hours' sleep.

In the morning, Kim was unable to tell who it was had been sobbing, as the people around were either sitting or standing.

The next night it was the same. The sobbing was louder. Again, Kim asked the man what the matter was.

"A problem shared is a problem halved," Kim said to the man. But the man would not speak. So again, Kim turned over on his mattress and tried to block his ears. On the other side, where it was lighter, a man who was obviously an inmate of long standing leered wildly at him. Kim shut his eyes, covering his ears with his hands. He tried to sleep but this time the noise of the sobbing with the fear of the half-mad, leering man on the other side kept him awake, so he got barely an hour's sleep.

But he had an idea what to do if it happened again.

The following night, when the sobbing started, Kim turned to the unhappy man. He had saved some water in his bottle, their daily ration, and now he offered it to the man.

"Come, friend, take a drink, will you? It'll calm your nerves and mind ..."

The man suddenly stopped his sobbing. "Thank you," he said, grasping the carafe and drinking down the remains of the water.

"Now tell me," Kim continued, "what is it that's causing this terrible nightly wailing? I know I'm young, but I've also seen great unhappiness and although I can't know what you know, or be who you are, I may have something useful to say about what is giving you so much pain."

"You are too young to have children so you cannot know the pain of leaving them ..."

"But I do know of the death of people you love and of leaving others because you must ..." He stopped a moment, hardly able to go on. "I'm only in prison because I tried to help a very nasty woman! Why are you here?"

"I've been here," said the weeping man, "for two years. I did nothing wrong except to cause the anger and envy of a local chief constable."

"How did you do that?" asked Kim.

"By practising my religion ..."

"What do you mean – he can't object to your prayers?"

"Oh yes! He objected to my prayers and the fact that every Saturday I would take my two little girls to the house of God and pray. 'Where's your wife?' he would ask. But I didn't answer him or tell him that my wife was working in a big house, doing cooking and kitchen work, and that she couldn't come with us during the day but only went to prayers at evening."

"But why are you in prison?"

"That chief constable. He started to spread stories about me. That I had another woman. That was the first story. Then he said I used to get drunk secretly. Then one day I was arrested. False charges. Well, you know what the courts are like, they send you down even when you're innocent of any crime. In my case they found something illegal in my pocket and gave me eight years. It was planted on me. I'd never seen it before and wouldn't even know what to do with it! But my wife, after all these stories, said she didn't know what to believe. She thought it must be true. She's a simple woman and she just thought it was impossible that a chief constable would lie. She thought I was the one who was lying. I've hardly spoken to her and now she's sent word she doesn't want to see me when I get out. She's looking after the children with the help of her sister and parents and doesn't want to see me any more."

"Only you haven't spoken to her," said Kim.

"No. She won't speak to me."

"Perhaps you should write to her. Explain what was happening with the chief constable. Tell her you love her."

"Explain? Write to her?" said the man, becoming distraught again. "Where do I get paper? How will I be able to get a letter to her from here?"

"I could take it. I should be out in a few weeks. I'll take it," Kim said.

"But what can I write on? They won't give me any paper or pencil!"

"Wait … look!" Kim searched around on the floor amongst the hay where they had their palliasses. "Look, here's a twig. There's plenty of dirt around …"

"What do you mean? Use the dirt to write with?"

"Yes," said Kim confidently.

"And what do I write on?"

"Ah, well, have you a … a … vest, yes! It's white. We can use that … Take it off and write on the inside of it! I'll put it on when I leave here. They'll never see it! They didn't even search me properly when I came in. They'll never search me going out. There's dirt all along the edge of the wall. You can start here. We'll roll it up each day. But think carefully before you write because there's not much space on it … What do you think? Is it a good idea?"

The man was now looking at Kim in wonder. "My name is Lullam," the man said, grasping Kim's hand. "My wife's name is Jisha and she works in the kitchens of a great house on the outskirts of Trasimid. The house is called 'Ardair'. When I've finished writing what I want to say, you promise you'll take it to her?"

"I promise," said Kim, shaking his hand and patting him on the head with the other. "Now you do that and let me have some sleep!" And Lullam immediately took off his vest and smoothed it over the bit of floor as he thought about what he was going to say.

Chapter 7
ARDAIR

After one month, Kim walked through the large, clanking gates out of the prison, blinking into the sunlight. He felt ecstatic. He could breathe without a stench coming through his nostrils; he could see the sun, the sky, the trees, the birds. The sounds were peaceful and delightful. Now perhaps, with care not to bump into anyone, or let anyone bump into him, he might have a better chance of finding Balquin.

There had been little light in the prison, apart from a few candles dotted around the large room all night. Even the exercise area was roofed in. But Lullam, working at night, had given Kim the finished letter written onto his vest and Kim had put it on and given Lullam his own vest to wear. Lullam had been worried that the mud he used to write the words would just crumble away and Kim promised he would go over it carefully with something indelible, so that his wife would be able to read it.

Waiting outside for him were Sabio and Bava in a little cart, pulled by Modo. Despite Kim's dirty and hungry appearance, he kissed them warmly and even gave Modo a hug.

"How are you?" Bava cried, so pleased to see her young lodger. "We have all been so worried. The prisons are terrible!"

"I believe you." Laughed Kim. "But I'm out now." Even Modo, happy to see him, gave him a kiss. Then they all set off for Tiésa's stall.

When they got there, Tiésa embraced the dishevelled-looking Kim.

"Glad to see you safe and sound."

"I'm so happy to be out. But I've done nothing – all this time wasted …"

"Only I've not wasted any time! I shall tell you later. Good news and bad news." She gave him tea to drink and sorted out clean but old clothes for him to wear, including a pair of trousers to make necessary adjustments into the waistband .

That evening a good meal was prepared. All the other lodgers were invited to dine and to listen to the sorry tale of Kim's arrest and near-execution, as well as the story of Lullam and his vest. Afterwards when the others had left and the remains of the meal had been taken away, Kim was left alone with Tiésa.

"Do you realise, I was going back to ask the blacksmith, Plosit, another question when that terrible woman knocked into me! I don't even know if I could find my way to the blacksmith's again now …"

"But I *have* been able to do some asking around," said Tiésa. "I have made enquiries about Balquin from your blacksmith, Plosit, and also about Aziel, the dead man you found. I can find no trace whatsoever of Aziel.

I think he must have come from another country. I even put a notice up in the town, but no-one replied. What I can't understand is what made you look under his boots! I would never have thought of it," Tiésa exclaimed.

"In my country, the anklet is a sign of wealth and carries identification, just the same as in my family we have a secret of sewing jewels into the inside of our waistbands for extra safety. That's how I found the diamond!"

"Maybe he comes from Strela, then," said Tiésa, mystified. "I just don't know. But regarding Balquin," she went on, "I have some interesting, if not completely good news for you."

"What is it?" asked Kim excitedly.

"Balquin changed his name to 'Camdovin'. A long time ago."

"Camdovin ...? And does he still live here in Trasimid?"

"He lives just outside the city. He was a blacksmith, it's true, but later he turned to trading and also to working on buildings and eventually he became a master builder."

"How extraordinary!"

"He is now a very rich man. He lives in a great house with a wife and family. He is considered one of the most eminent men of Trasimid, although I believe he is still only in his forties."

"This is amazing!" cried Kim.

"Yes, but listen ... The fact of his eminence also makes him very unapproachable, especially to you, a person who wants to remind him of a past he clearly wants to forget. He won't take kindly to a young man, even a prince, who calls him by his discarded name and who wants to know his most guarded secrets. We are going to have to think of a way round this … Money will have no effect on him. If he were still a blacksmith it would be different. But he is a wealthy man. He won't be easily tempted."

A wealthy man? Kim thought, amazed. How could that be when he used to be a kitchen boy? Perhaps a catastrophe in your life can lead to an advantage. Listening to Tiésa, Kim thought it could be true; but would Camdovin, this successful man, now want anything to do with a prince, only just turned sixteen years old, who was trying to remind him of his past?

Then, after a moment, Tiésa went on. "You're lucky you had the talisman. If you'd let that go, they'd probably have found you guilty of the robbery and executed you!"

Kim touched the top of his waistband nervously, feeling for the talisman.

"The only thing I can think of," Kim said tentatively, "is for me to find work in Camdovin's household."

"That's a possibility, but it's going to take a while, and you are going to have to use all your ingenuity."

"I have to do this," he said more determinedly. "I was thinking about all this in prison. I have to go on with what I started. But what could I do as a job there? I've only ever had servants myself!"

"Well, I presume you made yourself quite useful at Kelin's after you recovered from your fever? You're a clever chap; you will find the skills to make yourself useful to him. Because that's what it's going to take. He must get to know you and trust you. Ideally, he must find you indispensable. Then you might have a chance to ask your difficult questions. I suggest we invent a history for you so that at least you have a plausible reason for your travels here. You could say you came from Grailand."

"I could pretend, as I did with Kelin, that I must find my uncle in Memarn, because my father needs him to help build part of the house." Kim was buoyed up with the triumph of having at last discovered the whereabouts of the man whose secret he had to find out.

"Possibly … You have family in Grailand, where you studied a bit, but then came here. You'll have to find out if they need anyone to work at his house and what kind of work is needed there. We should adjust your history according to that."

So, the two of them worked out a story and the next day they went to the outskirts of the city, where Camdovin had a large house, called 'Ardair'. As soon as Kim saw the name of the house, he turned to Tiésa, almost whispering in disbelief and excitement, "This is the house where Lullam's wife, Jisha, works! I've not brought the vest with me because I was going to make the words clear for her in proper ink, but I will do that tonight. Perhaps she will be able to tell me if there's any work for me here."

"Let's try to find out more. Maybe someone in this market will know something."

At the nearby market they came to a stall with lots of

different cheeses. "What's that great house, over there?" Tiésa asked the stall holder.

"Oh that … That's Ardair, Camdovin's house," the stall holder answered.

"Who is he? He must be very rich."

"He's a master-builder. They say he's the finest architect and engineer of all Memarn but used to deal in horses. At the moment he's designing the prince's palace."

"The prince's palace! I thought the prince had a palace in the centre of the city!" said Tiésa.

"Oh, he does. But he wants another one in the countryside!" They laughed.

"How many servants does he have?" asked Kim.

"Who Camdovin? Ooh, I should say twenty, maybe. It's a big house."

"Don't suppose he needs servants now, does he?" Tiésa asked. "Only my grandson's been out of work for a while. He's a good worker, but his previous employer lost his position and had to dispense with many of his servants. So, since then he's had no work."

"I'm not sure. I know they've been looking for more staff … As I said, the master there is working on a new palace and I've heard he's taking on some new people. What kind, I don't know. You'll have to find out. Could be kitchen staff, gardening or cleaning – even building in the new place. Gardens are difficult at Ardair; people always leaving. I don't know why. You'll have to ask there."

"I can do cleaning or gardening!" Kim said quickly.

"I should go along and ask, then," the stall holder said.

"What?" asked Kim innocently. "Can I just go to the house and ask?"

"Yes. Why not?" The stallholder laughed.

"Thank you." And Kim turned to Tiésa. They bought some cheese and went to sit on a bench to eat it and drink water from a nearby well.

"I think it is better if *I* give Lullam's vest to his wife, rather than you," Tiésa said. "If you work at Ardair you can keep an eye on Jisha without her realising you know Lullam. You could have an influence on her, so that she becomes more reasonable towards him. And don't say too much about yourself. If it's a menial job they don't need to know much about you."

Kim decided to pretend he didn't care too much, not to look too desperate for a job there, although he really did want to get into that house somehow – whatever it took!

He went off and Tiésa sat waiting under a lemon tree. Kim found a side door to the house and pulled the bell. After a moment a man dressed in white jacket and grey trousers appeared at the door.

"Someone said you need a cleaner or kitchen worker or a gardener."

"Oh, yes. Possibly. Wait here a moment." And the man went off.

A minute later, he was back.

"Would you come in for a moment, please?"

Inside was a small hallway leading onto a series of stone-clad rooms, which led into one another. In the second of them sat two young men, eating at a table.

"This is the boy," he said to one of the young men. He turned to Kim. "Cleaning, you said?"

"Yes," said Kim.

"He wants a cleaning job. What do you think?"

"Just let me finish my lunch and I'll go and ask Mr Gralun."

After two more mouthfuls, the young man put down his fork and went out, while the other one kept eating.

A moment later, he was back.

"They've filled all the cleaning jobs. And there's nothing at the moment in the new palace, Mr Gralun says." He sat down and took another mouthful. "You might get a gardening job." He glanced at his companion. "You'd have to be pretty desperate, though. Melmed's difficult." He looked around him to make sure Melmed was not nearby. "We work for him in the gardens. He's very fussy …"

"Only has the best," said his companion, managing to look pleased with himself as well as having his mouth full of food.

"But," the first went on, "he can usually see people at six in the morning, so if you get here bright and early and be very nice to old Melmed, he might take you on. He's fussy, though," the young man repeated and laughed. "My name's Tordas, by the way. What's yours?"

"Kim."

"And this is Thovi," he said, indicating the other young man who was still eating. "See you tomorrow morning then. Come to the side door. Six o'clock."

* * *

In the morning at six o'clock sharp Kim was at the side door of Ardair wearing the same old, but clean clothes that Tiésa had given him when he came out of prison, and now desperately hoping there would be a job for him here. If there were no jobs in cleaning, he knew it might be the same story in gardening, though what you could see from the road was that the Ardair gardens were vast and full of great trees; they would clearly require a lot of work.

But when the door was opened by Tordas, his face showed failure.

"I think you'd better come back tomorrow at the same time," he said. "Melmed was in such a bad mood I didn't want to ask him about any gardening jobs. He would have bitten my head off and there definitely would have been no work. Maybe he'll be in a better mood tomorrow. The stupid thing is that he's in a bad mood mainly *because* there's too much work in the gardens. I know his nephew's coming to work here sometime. Not quite sure when." Tordas looked sheepishly apologetic as he closed the door and Kim walked away dejectedly.

What if there were no work tomorrow or when Melmed was in a good mood? He would have to think of some ruse to get into that house. He almost felt like watching the main entrance to see who came in or out, to perhaps get a glimpse of the man himself. How would he know if it were him? Would it be obvious who was the master of this house? Would Camdovin be followed by a retinue, as his father often was? Would he be surrounded by henchmen protecting him from unwanted people looking for work?

No. Wait until he found out whether he could actually have a job. Be patient, he thought – even though that was the last thing Kim felt.

So little time! There was the wise, young Sagesse probably about to be betrothed to some stranger; there was Pala, sad, morose and depressed at home with their father; there was his father's *Festival of the King's Rule* coming up at the end of next year and there was the ever-present threat of the curse hanging over Kim – hanging over them all – on and on into the future if Kim didn't finish his task and ask Balquin, now Camdovin, for the relevant documents. How could Kim be patient? But he had to be and would wait until tomorrow and not spy on the household until it became a last resort.

* * *

The next day, on his second appointment, Tordas greeted Kim with hope.

"He's in a good mood this morning." He winked. "Be nice to him and you might get a job helping us."

He led Kim through the corridor of rooms, into the dining area, where Melmed, in his late forties, a big gruff man with a beard, was finishing his coffee.

"This is Kim, sir, and he's very keen to work with us in the gardens."

Melmed glanced at Kim and grunted: "Know anything about gardening?"

"Well, I've worked my father's plot of land, planting vegetables and crops." Kim was thinking of Kelin and wished that in reality Kelin were his father.

"Plot of land, eh?" said Melmed gruffly. "I think you'll do." Then he turned to Tordas. "Get him some overalls, would you?" And turning again to Kim, "Start tomorrow morning? Same time?"

"Yes, sir. Absolutely." What a relief!

"You'll share a bedroom with Tordas and Thovi."

"Thank you, sir."

"You get forty crowns a month, plus bed and food, and every other Sunday off," Melmed said, now looking pleased.

At Tiésa's stall Kim was smiling and happy.

"That's wonderful," she said when he told her.

Kim couldn't stop smiling. "I can't believe it," he said again and again. "I'm actually going to be working in his house!" And his smile wouldn't go away.

"Do you get any time off?" asked Tiésa, when they were on their way back to Sabio's.

"One Sunday every fortnight."

"Good. We can meet then and find out how things are going."

"You've helped me so much, Tiésa. I don't know how to thank you."

"Well, it's a pleasure, my dear, but your work is by no means over, in fact it's only really just beginning, so keep your courage up."

In this way, Kim started as an under-gardener at Ardair.

* * *

At first the work was hard and tiring and it was all he could do to keep working all those hours. Prison had taken away the strength he had gained with Kelin and he was now having to build it up again very fast, without complaining about the pains he felt at night. But he enjoyed all the plants and the great gardens filled with beautiful trees.

On the first day, Thovi took him around the gardens.

"This is the lower garden. We have the rhododendrons here because of the moisture: azaleas, euphorbias and flowering hedges. At the higher points, over there," he said, pointing, "we have the cedars, which don't have much around them. Then over there, that hilly part, there are shrubs and hedges. Our vegetable garden is on the other side with a wall around it. You can just see the door to it in the wall, over there."

"I must confess – I don't know all the names of the plants and trees because I haven't had to deal with them before." Kim admitted.

"Don't worry. We'll show you what to do – and what not to do!" They both laughed. After that Thovi took Kim to the outhouses, where the garden equipment was kept.

"We must be clever with the vegetables," said Thovi, "because the house is vegetarian and needs fresh vegetables every day. And the kitchen staff deal with the animals – the goats and chickens for milk and eggs." He pointed to another area of the garden partly hidden by outhouses as they slowly made their way back to the greenhouse to get their orders from Melmed. "We don't have much contact with the other servants, even kitchen staff. We take flowers and vegetables for the house to the kitchens and the other servants hardly ever come down to the kitchens. Us gardeners are the lowest of the low!" He laughed.

Kim soon discovered that, with a two-hour lunch and siesta break at midday, they worked from six in the morning when it was light, until six every evening. After that, they bathed in the servants' baths, had some supper, chatted, played cards or chess or a kind of bowls and then went off to sleep.

As the days and weeks passed, Kim questioned Thovi and Tordas about his master and potential liberator, the great Camdovin.

"He is kind and generous and always has time for us if necessary," said Thovi seriously, as he weeded one of the flower beds

"What's his wife's name?" asked Kim digging around some plants.

"Atrell," Tordas said. "Everyone likes her. They have young children and two older boys are away. The eldest, Bertis, went to the east a year ago to trade in Sarquestan. The younger, Alman, is studying in Karmassos."

"Camdovin can be a bit abrupt. I mean, you don't approach him easily, do you?" said Tordas. Kim had seen him only twice from a distance and with no personal contact, he wondered how on earth he would get close to him.

"Do you never get to speak to him?" asked Kim,

suddenly panicked by this lack of contact with the man he so needed to question.

"Not really. I mean, what would we speak to him about? We hardly get to speak to, or even to see, the kitchen or house staff, let alone the master and his family. He always deals with Melmed on garden matters. Only with Melmed."

Kim looked daggers at Tordas, as if this young gardener were to blame. "That's crazy!" he exclaimed.

"What?" answered Tordas. "You're an under-gardener! He won't talk to you ... Anyway, what do you want to talk to him about?"

Kim shut up. He had gone too far. He didn't want it known that he had anything to say to Camdovin or to ask him. It was secret and must remain secret until the curse was known. He knew that, and he had let his temper run away with him. He looked down apologetically, not knowing what to say to the amiable Tordas.

"Sorry. I don't know ... nothing really ..." he said vaguely and turned away to do some cutting.

Then, one bright, sunny day when Kim was on his own in a little dip in the grounds, near to where the children played sometimes, a hard, leather ball came hurtling down just where he was working. It came smack into a ring of primroses and before Kim could pick it up, a young boy appeared.

"My older brother did that," he said. "Sorry."

Kim knew he must seize any chance he could, because soon Melmed's nephew would be taking over from him and Kim would have to leave Ardair.

"That is lucky!" he said. "It's landed in the middle of a posy ring …"

"Is it?" the boy asked. "I'll tell Tamis. He's the one who threw it."

"He must be a good thrower," said Kim.

"He is. But I don't think he realised how good!"

"What's *your* name?" asked Kim.

"I'm Didi, and that," he said pointing to a little girl who had just appeared from behind the same tall hedge, "is Gracia." The little girl came up to Kim and shook his hand seriously.

"And I'm Kim," said Kim, shaking her hand and then shaking Didi's hand. "Pleased to meet you. I work in the gardens. I expect I'll see you sometimes."

"Oh yes!" exclaimed Didi. "We often play out here. Ball games with the girls. Do you play? You could play with us!"

"Well, I do, but I don't think Melmed would take kindly to me not doing my work."

"Too bad," Didi commiserated. "I bet you're good at sports."

"I'm not too bad. Here." Kim picked the ball out of the flowers. "And remember this is lucky now!"

"Because," Didi went on, "we are going to have our annual ball game in two weeks. I would really love to have an older person on my team." Kim was surprised. He hadn't expected this.

"Wonderful," he said. "If I can get the time off gardening …"

"Oh, I'll arrange that with Zotos," Didi said and ran

off with his sister, waving. Kim heaved a sigh. At last! Contact with the family and, as it happened, Kim was quite good at sports.

*   *   *

A few days later, Tiésa made her way to the side entrance of the big house.

"May I possibly see one of the kitchen maids, Jisha?" she asked the person who opened the door. "I have something for her."

"Oh. Well, I can give it to her. She may be busy."

"I also have a message for her which I have to tell her and is private," said Tiésa quietly. "I don't mind waiting or coming back."

"I'll see if she's free. Wait here."

Two minutes later Jisha came to the side door.

"I am Jisha. Do you have something for me?"

"I have something from your husband."

"My husband, but …" Jisha put her hand to her mouth. "Come out here a moment." She led Tiésa outside, away from the door. "Is he ill?" she whispered.

"A friend of mine was in the same prison as your husband and managed to smuggle out a message written onto his vest. My friend said that Lullam is a good and kind man who has never been unfaithful to his wife and is in prison on a trumped-up charge." Tiésa handed Jisha the package containing the vest. "I haven't told anyone about it."

"Thank you," Jisha said anxiously, then grabbed the

parcel and ran back into the great house. "Thank you!" She repeated closing the door. Inside, she ran and hid the package in a tureen until she went to bed and could read it in private.

"My dearest wife," it read, "I am here in prison and have heard that you never want to speak to me again. But I have always loved you and our two daughters and I never could have done the things the chief law-officer said I had done. In the eyes of the law, a law-officer cannot lie. So, the judge assumed that I was the one who was lying. My friend who brings you this vest was almost executed for something he did not do. But he had an important character witness and was given a lenient sentence. I had no such witness. Please don't believe the chief law-officer's lies, but know that I have always told you the truth and I will love you and the children until I die. If I know you will speak to me when I get out, then living in this horror will be possible because I can hope to see you again. Your loving husband, Lullam."

Jisha's two roommates were woken several times that night by Jisha's sobbing. She just didn't know what to think any longer. Could she have been so wrong about Lullam? Had the chief law-officer lied? What about the things found in his pocket? Eventually she cried herself to sleep.

Chapter 8
AN IMPORTANT BALL GAME

On a spring day, about a week after Kim had seen the two children in the garden, and while Tordas, Thovi and Kim were eating their lunch with Melmed, Jisha ran in to their dining room.

"There's a message from Gralun," she said. "He says could Kim come and see him as soon as he's finished his lunch."

"Right-ho," said Kim casually, but excitedly wondering what it could be. "Thank you, Jisha. How are you?" he went on. Kim had made a point of being polite and friendly to her once he'd found out who she was.

"I'm well, but I must go on with the preparing!" she said. "Come and find me in the kitchen when you've finished and I'll take you up to him." Then she rushed off.

"Careful of her, she's a divorced woman!" teased Thovi.

"Not divorced …. just separated!" countered Tordas.

"Likes you though …" said Thovi.

"I hope no-one in the family's ill …" Melmed said mournfully. "That's the usual reason they call you up there. I suppose you'll have to have time off, won't you?" Melmed was extremely taciturn as well as a pessimist and he never really knew much about his gardeners.

"My family aren't in this country," Kim said, "so you needn't worry about that." He put the last mouthful into his mouth. "I'd only find out on my day off if there were anything wrong, and then I'd probably have to leave altogether!"

Kim went to clean himself up a bit and ten minutes later presented himself to Jisha, who took him up to a little room where Gralun, the servants' clerk, was sitting behind a desk.

"Kim …" Gralun said slowly.

"Yes, sir," said Kim.

"You'll be pleased to know your presence is requested next Sunday at a match, here at Ardair. Young master Didi has specifically asked for you because he says you're a wizard with a ball and he wants you on his team!" Gralun was smiling as he said this. "If it's one of your working Sundays, have it changed," he added.

"But I haven't got any suitable clothes …" Kim murmured.

"Don't worry. Some will be sent down. What size shoe?"

"Nine, sir." Then he asked, "Mr Gralun, will I have any time off on that Sunday?"

"You'll have the morning. It starts at two-thirty near the pavilion."

"Thank you, sir." Kim tried to hide his joy. Kim walked out of Gralun's office on air. At last he would have a chance to see the family in action and together. Maybe now he would even be able to speak to Camdovin.

The following Sunday Kim made his way early to Tiésa to tell her the good news and that his days off had been changed. He was always very careful when he went to see her because he had to cross the road where he had seen the men from his father's army. Kim often wore the clothes Kelin had given him but sometimes came out in the livery of Camdovin's household (a green top with black trousers for the gardeners) plus the old hat to hide his hair and face. Kim reckoned that dressed in his gardening livery he would also be quite hidden as it was obviously a servant's uniform; his father's army weren't looking for a servant, they were looking for a prince! And luckily, he hadn't seen any more of them. Maybe they'd given up. That would be wonderful, but knowing the general, it was unlikely he would ever give up. They had probably just moved on.

"And what are you like at sports?" Tiésa asked after he had told her the news. "Are you going to shame Didi's team or do them proud?"

"I've always done quite well at sports …" said Kim quietly, although he was more than excited at the prospect of the game. This might be his chance.

"Well, that's alright then, isn't it! I'll wait impatiently to hear what happens." She patted him on the back. "Courage!" she said and they laughed. "But take care …." she added, intently.

* * *

That afternoon, dressed in the clothes that had been sent over to him, and having adjusted the waistband in his trousers to accommodate the talisman, Kim made his way up towards the pavilion where the teams were gathering. It was mainly young boys, but there were a few older ones amongst them. One of them now came up to Kim and introduced himself.

"Hallo. I'm Nemesh. I've seen you in the gardens."

"How do you do. My name's Kim." They shook hands formally. It was strange how little he knew of upstairs. Working in the gardens, he saw few people because the servants rarely came down to the lower kitchens. When flowers were cut for the house, they were taken up by the under-maids. The gardeners didn't even eat with the kitchen staff, let alone the house staff.

"How come you're here then?" Nemesh asked.

"The young master, Didi, asked for me."

"Didi asked for you? I see. That's an honour. What did you do for that? Give him bowling lessons?"

"Not exactly …" Kim was surprised by Nemesh's slightly deriding tone of voice. "No. He just lost his ball and I gave it back."

At that moment the ten-year-old Didi, accompanied by another boy of the same age, came up to them.

"Hullo!" he said, smiling at Kim. "Glad you're here. This is my friend, Guz. I'm the captain of the team and we're bowling first. I'd like you to go second, Kim …"

"Well, Master Didi, I would …" and he hesitated. "But perhaps … Can I make a suggestion?"

"Yes, do!" said Didi.

"It might be better to have one or two strong bowlers later so that – you know – if anything happens at the beginning, you've got some good backup."

"Oh. I see." Didi turned to Guz. "What do you think, Guz. Good idea?"

Guz looked as if he had no idea.

"Why don't you try it, young master," said Nemesh. "Find out how good this gardener's advice is." Again, there was just the slightest tinge of a sneer.

"Yes! Okay, we'll do it that way. You can be ninth! How's that, Kim?"

"Very good!"

"Come and wait in the summer house. There are drinks and things to eat." Didi waved Kim and Nemesh over to the large pavilion where people were milling around.

"Nemesh!" Didi shouted as he went off. "I'd like you fourth!"

Nemesh waved acknowledgement and the two boys disappeared to find the team, as Kim and Nemesh walked over towards the summer house.

"How long have you worked here?" Kim asked Nemesh.

"Three years – God, it doesn't seem that long! Started when I was nineteen. It's all go, isn't it? You've probably found that out."

"We do work very hard," said Kim, thoughtfully. "On the other hand, it is a friendly place. I mean look – the family aren't unapproachable, are they?"

"You're one of the gardeners and you say it's a

friendly place! You must be getting on with Melmed!" Nemesh exclaimed.

"I like him, actually."

"No, when it comes to the children's matches, they're welcoming. A few servants are always included in those, but not much else. The master, Camdovin, hardly ever comes to these. Or if he does it's only for a quarter of an hour or so."

"And which is the mistress of Ardair?" Kim asked.

"You mean, you don't know who she is?"

"I've only been here barely a month and I've never seen her."

"Of course, you lot in the gardens have separate hours and separate tables, don't you? You probably don't know all the servants yet! And I've only ever seen you from the rooms when you've been doing gardens near the house."

"What's your job, then?" Kim asked him.

"I look after the two boys, Didi and his brother Tamis. I was valet to Bertis and Alman, but they're both away."

"Yes. I've heard they're abroad. So, show me where is the mother of all those children?"

"Why, here ..." Nemesh indicated a tall woman standing nearby with her back to them. Then he whispered: "This is she. Atrell is her name ..." The head of dark shiny curls turned suddenly, as if she'd heard, and Atrell gave a smile to Nemesh and a nod to Kim. She seemed to Kim to be too young to have six children, two of whom were grown up. He bowed to her, again wondering what kind of man was Camdovin. When he looked up again, she was talking to her neighbour, a giggling woman in a bright dress.

"And what's Camdovin like?" Kim asked quietly, curiosity getting the better of him. "What kind of a man is he? I've never seen him properly."

"Ah … He's a character."

"Is he friendly?" Kim needed more information about the man who held the key to his own secret.

"No. I wouldn't say that! Definitely not. He keeps his distance. He's a big character, has lived a lot. Came from humble beginnings and is proud of it, but never speaks about his past. He's a fierce man and handsome too. I say he's fierce – in fact I'm told he can show great kindness and gentleness to anyone in need. But he doesn't tolerate fools and that makes him bad-tempered at times."

"He sounds fascinating. Will I know him if he comes out for his quarter of an hour of watching his sons play?"

"He usually comes onto the balcony first to have a good look," said Nemesh. "Come on. Let's get some food. We can sit on the grass and watch." So Kim followed Nemesh and got himself a glass of lemonade and a cheese crunchie. The two of them now sat on the grass, chatting and watching the game. Kim was entranced. He looked at both players and the spectators, made up mainly of doting parents. He kept his eye on the balcony and watched Atrell with her children. The two little girls were like their mother and all of them dark. He was glad he was bowling late, because it would be more likely that Camdovin would come out before he played.

Nemesh went off to bowl his over and then came

Guz and Didi. As Didi was bowling – rather well, Kim thought – Kim suddenly saw the man on the balcony.

Camdovin was watching his son.

A moment later he had disappeared from the balcony and was striding out of the house, towards his wife.

Coming into view, he was not at all as Kim had seen from the distance. Not massive, not loud. He was striking nonetheless and smaller than he had seemed, fine featured, with eagle-eyes that took everything in. When his eyes moved over Kim, he stared hard at him for a moment as Kim looked away, not knowing how to react. Suddenly, momentarily, Kim thought that Camdovin knew why he was here.

The next moment there was a shout from the pitch.

"Kim!" It was Didi shouting and Kim's turn to bowl. He ran onto the pitch, his heart suddenly churning with nerves, but pretending that he did this every day. Now was the moment to make an impression. Also, although he had always been good at sports, it was a while since had played anything much. How rusty would he be? As he ran out, he sensed Camdovin watching him. Well, wasn't he watching all of them? Kim felt a peculiar sense that he must not let Camdovin down; that Kim must show him, prove to him how good he was, even if he was only a very young gardener, a newcomer and a nobody.

He bowled once, and then again. Both felt weak.

"A bit rusty …" Kim muttered to the referee standing behind him. On the third bowl he felt a surge of strength and saw it spin faster than the others. Wham! It seemed to go through the batsman straight onto the wicket.

A cheer went up and Kim laughed.

"Not so bad now!" exclaimed the referee to Kim.

The next batsman was out in two balls and the third was out in one. Kim was catching them out like ninepins.

Didi stood, cheering at the edge of the field. "Keep going Kim! Keep it up!" he shouted, with Guz clapping at his side.

Kim's bowling was getting into its stride and he had the feeling he could do anything. In all he had managed to get four batsmen out and, when amidst all the clapping, he ran off the field, Didi ran after him.

"Great bowling! How do you do it? Really brilliant!"

"I'll give you some tips, if you like. After the match."

"Yes please! I'll meet you in the summer house when it's over. I know a place you can show me …" Didi waved and ran off.

Kim ran up the slope towards the summer house. He needed a drink. To his right, amongst the spectators, he caught a glimpse of Camdovin, who eyed him again, smiling, as he passed. Should he stop and talk to him? But what could he say? He couldn't just blurt it all out, here and now. No. But he wanted to do so. He wanted to grab Camdovin and say, "I need your help! Please!" But Kim walked on, not daring to accost this formidable man.

When it was his turn to bat, Kim did almost better, eventually only being caught out after a hundred and seventy-four runs. Again, he walked off to clapping and pats on the back, flopping down onto a seat to watch the rest of the game.

Although Tamis was the elder of the two brothers, his

team was weaker. He had not thought to recruit as many of the servants and relied mainly on his school friends. Didi's team won easily and although Tamis shook hands with his brother at the end of the match, he was clearly in a temper about it.

Kim watched the two brothers for a moment, then got up and went to the summer house, helping himself to more food and a cold lemonade.

"Well done!" Nemesh said, approaching. "You're a fine player. Must have spent some time honing that bowling of yours!"

"Yes. We did it at school."

"What, in Grailand?"

"Yes. Why?"

"I didn't know they played these games there."

"They do. Not all over. But many schools have it and there are public matches," he said confidently.

"I see."

At that moment, luckily for Kim (who was on rather shaky ground regarding sports played in Grailand), Didi came up to him carrying a ball and bat.

"Come on, Kim! Eat up. I want you to show me your bowling!" He pulled Kim, food, drink and all, through a side door and ran to some trees at the back.

"Just in there …" Didi said, "a bit further on there's a clearing, we can – well you're the gardener, you must know the gardens!"

"Yes, I do …" Kim was trying to finish his mouthful. He put the remains on the grass outside the pavilion and ran after Didi, who had disappeared.

Didi was standing in a little clearing.

"Come on!" he shouted.

Kim took the ball. "What I do – and this is a trade secret, so don't go bandying it about! Most people pay me a fortune for this!" Kim was laughing now.

"I won't tell anyone!" Didi said emphatically. "I mean, I don't want the other team to win, do I?"

Now Kim showed Didi his special method with the ball, so that it seemed to very slightly change course. They tried it against the tree a few times.

"Look, Master Didi, you'll have to practise it. It won't come in just one day! It's taken me years to get it this good."

"And who did you learn it from?" asked Didi.

"That's my secret!" Kim laughed. "Come on, try again."

After twenty minutes Didi was obviously exhausted.

"I've had rather an exciting day. It's the first time my team's won over Tamis. Can I come and show it to you next week? I'll find you in the garden."

"Yes, that's fine as long as old Melmed doesn't catch us."

"That'll be alright. I'll tell him. And thanks," he added, as they moved towards the summer house. Kim breathed a sigh: contact at last, albeit with Camdovin's youngest son. It was certainly a big step in the right direction and he had really enjoyed the match!

* * *

The next day Tordas and Thovi teased Kim mercilessly about his sports prowess.

"We heard you done Didi's team proud!" said Tordas, weeding one of the flowerbeds. "They'll be taking you off gardens in no time and putting you up as valet to the boys!"

"I don't want to be a valet. Anyway, they've got one. Nemesh."

"Ah, yes, we all know about Nemesh," they joked. "He's been here a long time. Well in with the family, he is!"

Funny, thought Kim. I didn't think Didi liked him that much.

Tordas and Thovi soon stopped ribbing Kim about his sportsmanship. They got on with the work, planted bulbs, trimmed hedges, cut flowers for the house, dug, mowed, weeded and raked.

At the end of the day and exhausted, they cleaned themselves up and were sitting, being served supper. At that moment, Melmed came in, filling the doorway with his bulk. He glared slightly at Kim in his usual grumpy manner.

"Kim!" he said, "the master has asked me to make sure you have two and a half hours off twice a week to coach his sons at sports!"

Kim had just taken a mouthful. "What?" he exclaimed, spluttering.

"Yes. He was quite specific. He said his son, Didi, learned a great deal from you in a few minutes; he wants you to coach both the boys. You're to be there on Mondays and Thursdays from four in the afternoon to six."

"To be where, sir?"

"The summer pavilion. Starting this Thursday." And Melmed sat down at his place at the table and started to eat in silence.

"Didi really did take a liking to you, then!" Tordas exclaimed.

"Well! Our new sportsman!" Thovi said, thumping Kim on the back and making him splutter again.

That night, Kim wrote a letter to his sister, hoping against hope that his father wouldn't get wind of it:

Dear Pala, I have at last found the person I've been looking for. But please do not say anything to Father as I believe he has men looking for me. This letter is being sent by a friend who goes away from where I am every two weeks to sell his wares in a town nearby. You must not know where I am, in case Father's men get hold of this letter.

The man is well-known here. He is wealthy and prominent and I am over-awed as to how he got to where he is. I am working in his house at the moment. Of course, no-one here knows who I really am and I want to keep it that way until I have found out what I need to know. With my friend, who has a stall, we have worked out a history for me so that the people I work for do not know where I really come from. It's hard work, but they're going to chuck me out soon as my boss's nephew takes over from me. It was arranged long before I got here. I am hoping against hope that there will be another job for me here.

I miss you. I miss Cal also. Do go and see him if you can. I know he's fond of you and he really is a good person to talk to. I also miss Sagesse. You know how much I care about her.

She's always in my thoughts and I am terrified her mother will get her betrothed to some horrible stranger before I get back. It all seems to be taking far too long and I've not even had a conversation with the man yet. It's difficult, but it's important I play my cards right. Luckily, I played in a ball game here and the master wants me to coach two of his children in sports. Well, you know I'm quite good at that, so I may get closer to him that way. He's not an easy man to talk to, though, and I couldn't just go up to him and say I need to talk to him. He'd probably send me away immediately. I must find a way to get his trust, but at the moment I've just no idea how I'm going to do that.

Say hullo to Cal. Tell him I really missed him when he left and almost rode back to get him to come with me. But then I thought I ought to be brave enough to do this difficult thing on my own, as Mother said I should.

I hope you're not having too terrible a time at the castle. I am coming back as soon as I can. I love you and am thinking of you.

Your brother,
Kim

He went on thinking about Pala, and how serious she had been when he had last seen her. He had never really shown how fond he was of her because he had been so intent on his own problems. And she had become more and more distant and silent, although her sadness at their mother's death was obvious. Now he missed her terribly and wished that she was safe with him in Trasimid, in Ardair even. Somehow, Ardair seemed so much safer than Koremine Castle. And, since seeing his father's men – who *must* have been looking for him – Kim had a new fear: that his father would disinherit him if he found out what Kim was doing.

Chapter 9
THE LOST SON

Suddenly, Kim was now sports coach to the two boys, whom he found to be bright and quick, and he was soon able to coach them in all the sports he knew.

As Kim arrived at the pavilion for their practice one day, he found Camdovin there with Didi and Tamis.

"Good afternoon," Camdovin said.

"Sir …" was all Kim could get out. He was completely taken aback by this unexpected presence.

"I hear you're a master sportsman," Camdovin went on.

"No, not really, sir. I was just good at sports at school, and I haven't forgotten them. We had a good teacher."

"Where was that?"

"Grailand, sir. Derkia."

"Grailand, I see. You've come quite far then. Is it your plan to stay in Memarn?"

"I'm happy here, yes sir. I may return one day to my home, but at present I am content."

"And what else did they teach you at your school? Languages? History? Geography?"

"Well, yes sir. The usual," he lied. "I mean … I don't understand …"

"I have reason to ask you. My two younger sons like you, they learn well from you and they need some coaching in school work. I want them to get a first-class education. I never had such chances, myself. I wondered whether you have a knowledge of all the subjects?"

"Well … yes sir. I had a tolerable schooling. My teachers were pleased with me. But I didn't pursue my studies. I wanted to travel."

"I would like you to show them how best to go about doing their homework. Not to do it for them, you understand, simply to point out what they have to do – then they must do it."

"Yes. I … I think I could do that. Do you have a library they could use, if necessary?"

"Yes," answered Camdovin, smiling broadly. "We do. Funny kind of a gardener, you are, asking me if I have a library!"

"I'm sorry, sir. I just thought it might be easier …"

"No! You're right! Look, let's make it every afternoon from five o'clock for three hours. In the mornings you can prepare lessons or do some clerical work in Gralun's office. You can eat supper with the children, and Gralun will see to new clothes for you and give you a new roommate – probably Nemesh. Gralun will tell you exactly where you'll be. Go and see him."

"Right."

"And I want regular reports from you."

"Yes, sir."

"Good luck." With that Camdovin left them and strode off down the slope, towards the house.

Kim, still in a daze said, "Well! Let's get on, shall we? Show me your bowling!"

* * *

"Things are progressing well." The delighted Tiésa smiled when Kim next saw her. "You're doing absolutely the right thing, my boy. Getting there slowly. And he was friendly, you say, Camdovin?"

"Very friendly and not at all fierce."

"Then you're in with a good chance. Keep your ears open. You will have to prove yourself to Camdovin in a special way."

"What do you mean?" asked Kim.

"I mean he is not to be trifled with. If you want him to give you the information he has fought all his life to conceal – to deny even – then he will have to feel you are uniquely trustworthy and utterly genuine, so that he wants to assist you. This will take careful words and careful actions."

"I do feel bad," answered Kim. "In a way, I mean. I feel maybe it's not right, what I'm doing. I'm deceiving him in some ways, aren't I? Do I have the right to do this?"

Tiésa looked at him gravely. "I think – however difficult it is – you have no other choice. If he knew why you were here, he would probably dismiss you on the spot. But you're not actually doing anything wrong. You have to be patient and hope that the right moment will present itself."

"The trouble is, I haven't got that much time, have I?"

He turned away from her in pain and inspected some of the herbs in front of him. "I haven't the time to wait for this 'moment', as you put it."

Tiésa went inside her cubby hole behind the stall. She knew that young people were impatient, that was natural. But there was something else eating at Kim and she didn't know what it was. She made him some tea, watching him from inside, wondering what that something was.

When she brought out the tea, they drank in silence. "Tell me what happens, won't you?" she said kindly, as Kim finished his tea and went off.

"Of course, I will," he said. But he was distant and preoccupied as he turned to go back to Ardair.

* * *

Kim now started his homework-tutoring and after a month the two boys were flourishing.

"How's it going?" Nemesh asked one evening when Kim, laden with books, got back to their shared room.

His relationship with Nemesh had been slowly turning sour for some time. Nemesh had realised long ago that Kim, young though he was, had outclassed him in the servant-hierarchy race, and he didn't like it. All the same, Kim tried to keep on good terms with his roommate.

"It's going well, I think," said Kim modestly. In fact, he knew it was a success and the boys were doing well. "I'm exhausted, though," he said truthfully, as he flopped down onto his bed. "Intelligent children aren't easy!" Kim laughed.

"They take it out of you, don't they?" agreed Nemesh.

"In a nice way, of course ..." Kim responded. "You're up late, aren't you?" Usually, Nemesh was asleep if Kim was late; the valets had to get up early in the mornings.

"Listen," Nemesh went on, in gossip mode. Nemesh did love to gossip. "Everyone's worried."

"What do you mean 'worried'? What about?" asked Kim.

"Well, you know that Alman is away in Karmassos, studying science?"

"Yes. I knew that."

"Well, Bertis has been trading abroad but has not contacted the family for three or four months," went on Nemesh.

"I didn't know that."

"Actually, that alone is not too bad," Nemesh continued. "Bandits have been roaming around for years, messing with postal services. A lot never arrives."

"He may have been writing but it was stolen by bandits? Is that what you mean?" Kim wondered about his letter to Pala. Would that have been stolen?

"Well, the family didn't know and were in two minds and quite worried; and then one trader, who should have met up with Bertis in Etarm, came back saying he hadn't met up with him and hadn't seen him for four months. So then there was panic. But yesterday, a friend of Camdovin just returned from abroad said he saw Bertis in Lorthal just a few weeks ago. They didn't speak because Bertis was at the other end of the hall, surrounded by people. But there was absolutely no doubt it was Bertis."

"So, everyone's mind has been set at rest," said Kim quietly, trying to imagine what Camdovin's eldest son was like. He was glad that everything was okay with Camdovin and Atrell's eldest. It would be more difficult for Kim to work out how to approach Camdovin if his family were in a turmoil. He felt, now that things were going so well with the two youngest boys, that he was near to having a heart-to-heart talk with his master; he just had to choose the right moment.

The two young boys now became Kim's life, although he himself was not much older than they were. He knew practically everything about them, more now even than did their valet, Nemesh. He also came into contact with their mother, as Atrell occasionally entrusted the little girls to him for tuition. Kim was often seen hurrying along corridors to get to Camdovin's library, to find the right books for their study, as well as helping out in some secretarial or clerical work that needed to be done for the household.

Sometimes Camdovin, always friendly and courteous, arrived at the end of a session to discuss his sons' progress.

"How are they getting on? Are they behaving themselves?" Camdovin joked, knowing that two little boys together can be quite a handful.

"Yes. Behaving well and keen also," Kim answered.

"Didi's stories are very good now. Interesting and well-written. And Tamis got a ninety percent mark in his maths test."

"Glad to hear it." Camdovin gave Kim a handshake and was off.

Although Kim felt impatient, it still wasn't the time to collar his master and tell him the real reason he was here. He had been warned by Tiésa to bide his time, but it was getting more and more difficult as time itself was dwindling; he feared the curse and its possible worse disaster, and he was ill at ease with the kind of deception he was perpetrating on Camdovin and his children, which, although not harming them, felt uncomfortable.

One day, visiting Tiésa on some time off, always carefully covered with his hat and on the lookout for his father's men, Kim was choosing a bit of fruit to buy. Some voices wafted towards him, catching his attention. He looked round and saw two older men, who looked like town officials.

"So, how did you get on in Beran?" said one to the other.

"Yes, very well," said the other, wiping sweat from his brow. "It's certainly cooler there than here." He laughed. "King Ambab's doing well, always amiable and good tempered. Such a pity his eldest daughter's so ill."

"Yes, Sagesse. I heard. What's wrong with her then?" asked the first man.

"Well, no-one knows exactly and they can't find a cure for her, though they've tried all the physicians they can find in Beran."

What was Kim hearing? My God, wasn't this further proof of the power of this curse? And every day he was here, he was losing time where he could be solving the mystery of the curse; every day was allowing the possibility of new problems emerging. What if Sagesse died? He didn't dare think of anything like that, and yet it was a possibility that the girl he thought of nearly every moment of the day, her smile, her gentle laugh and her bright intelligence would suddenly, like his mother, not be there anymore.

At the same time, it was crucial that he talk to Camdovin at the right moment so as not to frighten the great man into turning him away. He would have to bide his time, Kim thought miserably. There was nothing else to do.

A week later, on the way from the study room, Kim met Jisha in the corridor.

"Hullo, Jisha!" he exclaimed, taking the chance to chat with her. He had thought a lot about poor old Lullam, incarcerated for no reason. "How's it going?"

"Oh, I've got too much work, as usual, and I really would like to get away from this lovely house at times." She laughed.

"This house is heaven compared with some things I've seen," Kim ventured, wondering how secure any 'secret' would be with Jisha.

"Why? What have you seen, then? Bad things?"

"Well, yes." Kim's voice quietened. "Don't tell anyone this, but I was actually once thrown into prison for something I had not done ..."

"Really? What, for no reason?" Jisha was shocked.

"It was a terrible thing for me! A woman lied to save her own skin and I had actually been trying to help her."

"My God! How terrible …"

"It was. Really terrible. So, believe me, this place is heaven."

Jisha laughed, but underneath there sneaked a worry. "I didn't know that people could be put into jail for no reason."

"They can." And, with a wave, Kim left her, hurrying off to the library, pleased that he may have sown some doubt in her mind.

*   *   *

A few days after that, when Kim arrived at the appointed hour, he opened the door to the study room to find both Didi and Tamis looking dark and solemn.

"Whatever is the matter?" he asked, mystified.

"It's just that we've had some bad news," answered Tamis, cautiously.

"Oh dear …" Kim would wait for them to tell him if they wanted. "I hope it won't interfere with our studies. Studying can be a great antidote to bad news, you know," he said calmly.

"What's an antidote?"

"A kind of cure: if you have bad news and it's painful, studying and work can take away some of that pain."

"It's to do with our brother …" Didi let out.

"Oh …" Kim waited. "Bad news?"

"We're not sure. It could be."

"Well do you want to tell me about it or shall we put it out of our minds for now?" Kim was curious but he wouldn't show it.

"We'll get on with some work," said Tamis.

"Good. Only if it's very important we should probably talk about it. What have you got today?"

"I've done my history essay, but I need some help with geometry."

The three of them worked solidly, quietly and steadily for an hour, and then less steadily for the rest of the time. By eight o'clock Kim was worn out.

Later, when he got to his room, he found the valet in a state of excitement.

"Did they tell you?" Nemesh immediately asked Kim.

"Erm … well they said they were very upset …" Kim responded, guardedly. He was still cautious with Nemesh and certainly did not mention to Nemesh his talks with Camdovin and Atrell about their sons: Nemesh would probably have had a heart attack.

"He seems to have disappeared!" Nemesh spoke with some triumph.

"Oh … you mean …!"

"Bertis!" Nemesh went on. "No trace of him! Apparently Camdovin sent out some scouts to make sure he had seen the people he was supposed to have seen. It seems more than four months since anyone's seen him! It's terrible! Camdovin's gone into a depression. Alman, the second son's been recalled from Karmassos. They've no idea what could have happened!"

"Was he on his own?"

"No. That's just it! His aide has not been seen either. Lundell, a great big man on a fast, little horse. They think the man Camdovin's friend saw at the party must have been someone who looked like him."

This was depressing news. The family were a close, loving family; they would now be in a state of gloom.

"And the authorities can't do anything," said Nemesh. Again, Kim heard the note of triumph. "They never do. They are more worried about their little wars than with bandits and robbers who overrun our country disrupting all the services. The postal service has been in chaos for a long time because of robbers; travel's disrupted; trade's unsafe. Camdovin intends to go to search for Bertis himself, and he is taking a specially selected group with him."

Kim walked to the window in dismay. Outside, the gardens were still and bright in the moonlight. There was a difference: none of *his* family knew where he was, although he had written one or two letters home. Even Pala had no idea exactly where he was. But he had made clear he would not contact her or their father. Bertis, though, had no reason to hide where he was travelling.

This was going badly. If Camdovin was away, how could Kim get closer to him? He was already closer than most in the household. How would he be able to prove himself so that the master would reveal to him a secret that he had so carefully kept hidden? What would Kim have to do to be able to ask Camdovin about the quarrel? These thoughts and questions plagued Kim incessantly, like a gnawing ailment – yet again and again he feared spoiling the relationship he had with his master.

"What is it?" murmured Nemesh, surprised as Kim turned towards him, his face distraught. "What's the matter?"

"Oh … all this. It's terrible," Kim answered vaguely.

Nemesh gave a sniff and got into his bed. "Yes, it is rather terrible, I suppose," he said turning over, away from Kim.

But Kim felt despairing. How would he be in time to save Sagesse from her illness and her mother's plans? Suddenly he was overcome with a frightening feeling that all the time he had spent here could come to nothing at all.

* * *

The next day the household despondency was palpable. In the afternoon Kim had difficulty in getting his two students to do a thing.

"It's very important we try to do some work. Really!" He had been hearing from the two boys about the disappearance of their older brother, but now he was losing patience with them, as they were not getting any studying done.

"I have decided something …" Tamis declared eventually, eyeing Kim with a challenging look.

"And what is that?"

"I have decided to go with Father and the search group."

"Do you think he'll take you?" asked Kim.

"Well, if he doesn't want me to go with him, I shall follow them anyway." Tamis glowed triumphantly. He had worked everything out.

"I'll come too," said Didi, less certainly.

"I'm not sure that's a good idea," ventured Kim, not wanting to hurt their clearly upset feelings about all this.

"No. I don't care …" said Tamis. "I just want to help find my brother."

"Anyway," Kim added, "what about your mother. She needs you two by her at this time." The two boys fell silent. "Your father will need you to stay …"

"She doesn't need us …" Didi said weakly.

"At such a time she will need you greatly!" Kim looked at them squarely.

"Well, what do you think, Tamis? Perhaps we should stay?" Didi said.

"I want to find my brother … I don't care whether my father wants me to go or not. I'll go after them in secret!" Tamis repeated, defiantly.

"That would not be a good thing to do." Kim knew how Tamis felt but, knowing the dangers, he had to dissuade him. "We can discuss it tomorrow." The boys picked up their books and shuffled out of the room in disarray, as Kim pensively tidied up. Today's session had not gone well, but perhaps the boys might come to a sensible plan tomorrow rather than just to follow their father; Camdovin would surely not allow them on the search.

Kim had nearly finished when Atrell came into the room. She closed the door quietly behind her and sat down on one of the chairs.

"I suppose you must have heard by now the state we're in about my eldest son?"

Kim remained standing, surprised at this unexpected visit. "Yes, my lady. I'm very sorry about it. You must all be extremely worried."

"We are. And I think Didi and Tamis are also."

"In fact, we've just been having a conversation about it," Kim said. Atrell looked expectantly towards him. "I wonder if it would be possible to have a word with both you and your husband about what they said." Kim was not in the habit of telling tales, but in this case, he thought it was serious.

"Of course. They're distressed, like all of us. We'll go to his study now."

Kim followed Atrell along the corridors until they reached Camdovin's study. She knocked loudly and went in.

"Please come in," she said to Kim, who hesitated.

He had heard about this wonderful study where the master often sat for days on end, reading, working on designs and making up for what he called his lack of education. Kim knew it had been beautifully decorated with exotic colours and leaves of gold, and that at night great lamps shone in the room, lighting up the whole garden on that side. And he knew that during the day the windows allowed the sun to fall onto the room so that it seemed to glow. Now he entered the great chamber.

"Let's sit over here," said Atrell, going off towards a sofa and chairs at the side of the room. "It's more comfortable."

Camdovin shook Kim's hand and they all sat down. Kim felt awkward, sensing the anguish of both parents about their son. So much in Kim's life depended upon an improving relationship with Camdovin. Atrell helped him out.

"Something Tamis and Didi said, Kim thinks you should know about."

"What is it?" Camdovin looked even more worried.

"Well, sir … Please understand, I don't want to lose their trust."

"That would be difficult. They trust you very much," Camdovin said.

"Or to feel I have betrayed their trust by saying this."

"I can assure you, neither I nor my wife will mention it."

"Thank you, sir. Well … I think they're feeling it a lot. All this about your son, Bertis. They told me that you're intending to go and search for him."

"When I have arranged it all."

"The trouble is that Tamis wants to come with you. He is determined to help you find Bertis. Didi also. But Tamis says he'll follow you even if you forbid him to come. I said I thought he would be needed at Ardair. That his mother would need support …" Kim turned to Atrell. "I hope I wasn't wrong in saying this; I had to say that you would need them – with your husband not being here."

"You did right," said Camdovin. "I will definitely talk to them, perhaps entrust them with caring for the family while we're away. You've spoken well. Thank you." He got up and shook Kim's hand again. "Didi was right," he said quietly. "You are a valuable person to have in my household."

Kim left them with a glow of gratitude that Camdovin had shown his strength by listening to a youthful and lowly servant. It wasn't all worthless. Yet although Kim was getting somewhere with this complex, secretive and appealing man, clearly now, with his son missing, it was not the moment to talk. When would that moment be? Sagesse was ill; his own father had soldiers searching for him and would soon have his *Festival*; and things, without the knowledge he needed, would get worse in his own family and throughout the land: time was pressing.

The upshot was that three days later, a day before he and his party were to leave on their search, Camdovin asked Kim to bring his two younger boys to him.

"Listen," Camdovin said after both Atrell, Kim and the two boys had taken seats on the study sofas. "You know how very worried we both are about Bertis. We have made inquiries and searches and nothing has been heard at all. We are not even sure where he's travelled, because he is in the habit of travelling all over the place. No-one has seen him or his aide, Lundell, for many months. It's a mystery and one which – somehow – I hope to solve."

"Are you going to travel all over the place?" asked Tamis.

"We might have to. There are two strands of work that are essential now. One is the search itself, for Bertis and Lundell, which I am making with a small party and which could take up to a month. The other is here at Ardair, where I need you both, especially Tamis, being older, to take on as an equally important duty: the task of keeping Ardair safe and free from trouble. As Tamis knows, Alman – who is back from Karmassos – is coming with me on the search so that you, Tamis, will be in charge here, together of course with your mother."

Both boys were now looking very serious and slightly chastened.

"What? Us in charge?" said the surprised Tamis.

"If anything very important comes up, of course there is my trusty old Etsas and then Gralun, who can take over, if necessary." Camdovin turned to Kim. "Etsas looks after the horses and has been with me for very many years. I trust him with my life." He turned back to the boys. "You must continue with your studies under all circumstances; but what I especially need is for you to help your mother maintain calm here at Ardair, and if something really serious happens while I am away, you must contact your uncle in the south. But I do need both of you, Tamis and Didi, to maintain the quiet peace while I am away. That is almost as important as the success of the search." Camdovin stopped and looked intently at his two youngest sons. "Are you happy with all this?"

Tamis and Didi looked at each other and nodded seriously.

"And we have agreed that Mother will have reports from Kim as to how you are doing in your studies."

The two boys nodded again, sheepishly, but grateful that their risky plan had now been put out of action.

A day later, the party of twelve left and, although Atrell and the two little girls cried, Didi and Tamis remained serious, as Kim battled in his mind with the confused frustration and disappointment he felt at Camdovin's departure.

* * *

"But you're doing a magnificent job!" Tiésa asserted when he voiced his fears to her.

"What if he's away for more than a month?" Kim moaned. "It could still take ages to get close to him." He had not told her about Sagesse and his terrible fear about her illness.

"If it's Kelin you're worried about, you know he will be at the well in the City of Towers every year for several days. But maybe it's something else …?" Tiésa was silent for a moment, then went on. "I don't want to pry, but I have a feeling there's something else worrying you."

"Is there?" Kim lied.

"I've noticed this before. Something's on your mind and possibly making this task more difficult," she insisted gently.

Tiésa, Kim knew, wouldn't go on at him if she didn't think it was important. It was all too distressing and pre-occupying and he knew he needed her wise words. So he relented. "It's a person I'm worried about …" Kim said, quietly.

"A person? Who, then?" asked Tiésa.

"A friend. A girl I've known since I was a child."

"A girl, I see. And may I know her name?" pursued the herb doctor.

"Her name's Sagesse and she's the daughter of King Ambab, of Beran."

"I see. And you love her?"

"Well, I can't get her out of my mind, if that's what you mean," said Kim worriedly.

"Is there something wrong, then?"

"Yes." He paused, staring at the ground. "Two things … First, I'm scared her mother will get her betrothed to some rich stranger before I get back in time." He stopped again.

"And second?"

"I heard someone in the street saying they had been in Beran recently. He said that Sagesse is very ill and they can't find a cure."

"Ah, I see," Tiésa hesitated. "That's difficult. But, tell me, what's worse: to rush off to Beran, trying to cure her with no means at your disposal, or to have talked with Camdovin and be able to go to Beran with some success behind you? If you go to her now, you will have no real way of helping her; if you go with the documents or papers that you hope for from Camdovin, you have a good chance of helping her."

"I actually think this curse is the cause of her illness," ventured Kim.

"Well, there you are, then! You, having got rid of the curse – or well on the way to doing so – have some chance of *really* curing her. Because when an evil deed is known about by everyone, and possibly a punishment given to the wrongdoers, it also gets rid of the evil effects of the curse. They somehow disintegrate and have no further power. But without solving the overriding problem of this curse, it is my belief that Sagesse, your dear friend, will only get worse. That is what I think, anyway. Mull it over, my dear. Without the papers you are hoping to get from Camdovin, you will have nothing to help her with. Although," she went on, "if I knew what was wrong with her, I might know which herbs could cure her, or at least help her. But we don't know, do we? So, I recommend that you talk to Camdovin before running off, empty handed, to your princess."

Kim sat silent for a moment. Tiésa always talked such sense, and he didn't know what to say in response.

"You're right, of course," he said eventually, getting up from the stool he'd been sitting on and looking over the multitudes of herbs and spices: Tiésa's cures. "Thank you, Tiésa," he said, touching her hand. "Thank you. I'll try to be patient." And he walked slowly away, towards Ardair, pulling his hat carefully down over his head.

Then a picture of Sagesse came into his mind as clear as daylight. He watched her until the picture faded away. He spoke her name silently and wished to be near her, wished for that feeling of oneness when they were with each other, because they had been close all their lives and there was not a strange thing about each other. But he had terrible fears for her now, with the thought that the curse was affecting her life as well.

* * *

At Vocimere Palace, in the country of Beran, with its lush hills, forests and lakes – a country ruled by King Ambab – Princess Sagesse lay on her bed, seriously ill.

"I don't know what is wrong with her," Queen Flura moaned to King Ambab. "The physicians cannot agree."

"We'll find another physician. Abroad, if necessary," said the king.

"She still isn't eating properly. In fact, she says she feels sick most of the time. And I don't know how to get her to eat. None of them know what's wrong and she often seems to be in pain."

"We shall do absolutely everything possible," the king said, agonised. Both were beside themselves with worry.

"I think it's past stories," the queen said firmly, as if that made any sense; as if that statement could clarify the matter of Sagesse's illness.

"I've no idea what you mean. Did something happen that you know about?"

"No. Nothing that I know about. But I must take her some food …"

"Her maid can bring her food. You don't have to do that." The king was at a loss. Why was the queen behaving like a serving maid?

But the queen persisted and when she got to Sagesse's rooms, the maid let her in and she took the bowl of soup to her daughter.

"I want you to eat all that soup. After that I'll bring you some books to read. They might make you feel better. Flower arranging is also good."

"No, Mother. I don't want you to bring me books, and wonderful though flower arranging can be, I would prefer paper and pen," Sagesse protested. "I love flowers, but not at the moment. I just want to sleep. Please leave me alone … I don't want to see anyone!"

"Oh dear …" And the queen left, upset that she was being shunned by her own daughter.

Sagesse refused most of her food and spent her time drawing her garden from her window and writing poetry; these were the things keeping her alive. All this now became a way of life for King Ambab and his family. They started to get used to Sagesse's new ways and, for a time, as Sagesse sat in her room gazing out over the park which surrounded the palace, the forces that had buffeted her, pushing and pulling her into unknown directions, started to subside and she felt calmer.

But as time went on, Sagesse started to feel again the old pains, the terrors coming back at her as if by some power that had nothing to do with her life here. She knew that Kim had set off on his travels and that he might be away for a while, but now, after months and months, there was still no news of his return.

Chapter 10
AN EXTRAORDINARY REALISATION

Kim was still struggling to keep all the strands of life at Ardair from clashing and causing him and others difficulties.

With Camdovin away, part of Kim felt his presence as tutor was meaningless. He had not come all this way in order to be a tutor. At the same time, if everything continued smoothly with the family, despite the anguish, he knew he might get closer to Camdovin; it could be the time for him to prove himself. Whatever the outcome of Camdovin's journey, maybe he would in some way be grateful that he had helped to hold the fort while he was away?

The next Sunday, Kim arrived back earlier than usual from visiting Sabio, Bava and Tiésa and he sat in the garden outside the kitchen, marvelling at the great trees. Jisha saw him arrive, brought out some tea and said she would sit with him for a few minutes.

"Tell me about your time in prison," Jisha said, after a moment. "Was it in Trasimid, or somewhere else?"

"Far away to the west, the town of Lorthal," Kim lied.

"And what happened?"

"A woman swore that I had tried to steal her purse because she bumped into me and I ran after the thieves who stole it from her … And I can assure you I met a few other people in prison who were completely innocent of any crime. It was horrible for them because sometimes their family didn't believe they were innocent." Kim went silent, waiting. Jisha had never mentioned Lullam. Now Kim sensed the conflict going around in her head.

At last she took courage and asked: "But what if a chief law-officer says they are definitely guilty? Then they must be, don't you think?"

"Well, not necessarily. If my brother – if I had one – were convicted on the say-so of a law-officer, I think I would have to find out something about the law-officer before believing him: if he is an honest man or not. I wouldn't believe him just because he was a lawman. Especially if my brother was honest."

Jisha suddenly rushed back to the kitchen to get more tea. When she came out again, there were red rims round her eyes.

"It's not as simple as that …" she said quietly.

Kim was silent. He thought he could be more effective if he seemed to know nothing. So eventually he said: "Well, thank God it was a long time ago because prison's a horrible place to be …" Then he got up. "Thanks for the tea, Jisha." And he left her to mull over his words.

Coming from the kitchen, he met Nemesh, who had seen them.

"Nice, isn't she?" he said.

"Who?" Kim asked, surprised.

"Jisha, of course," Nemesh said.

"Jisha? Yes. She's lovely! One of the prettiest!" Kim answered Nemesh as casually as he could. He was used to the banter that went on and he was used to Nemesh's leading questions. Anyway, it was true; Jisha was one of the prettiest of the servants, but Kim had other things on his mind.

"And why were you so late last night?"

"What kind of question is that?" Kim kicked himself for not realising where all this was leading.

"I heard you come in past one o'clock."

"Yes. I was working late. What's wrong with that?" Kim rapidly felt his fury taking over. "I was working late!" he repeated, but he was now ready to lash out at Nemesh.

"I can see, you know! I'm not blind!" Nemesh hissed at him.

"See what? Me! In the library!" Kim suddenly felt he was losing control of himself. He wanted to punch Nemesh but he somehow realised that if he started a fight here, it could have disastrous effects in the delicate situation the whole house was in at the moment. "I don't know what you're trying to say!" Kim spat out at Nemesh and with that he got up and left him.

* * *

Now Kim stopped speaking to Nemesh because he seemed to take everything the wrong way and Kim felt sure that whatever he said would lead to trouble.

Reluctantly, he went to see Gralun to find out if he could change rooms.

"Why?" asked Gralun.

"Nemesh … He is being very difficult. I really don't think he likes me at all …" Kim said finally.

"Well," said Gralun. "If it's that difficult you can share with Trigan, on the first floor at the back. Trigan couldn't go with the search party."

So Kim moved rooms that night to another part of the house.

The next day Kim got lost on his way to the study room. He found himself in unknown corridors and came to a wide double staircase which he had never seen before. He decided to go back and start again, taking a longer way round, which he knew. When eventually he arrived in the study room, the boys were arguing,

"It's not 'Adzil' it's 'Aziel'!" Tamis was saying.

"No, I remember, it's definitely 'Adzil'!" retorted Didi.

"And who is Adzil or Aziel?" asked Kim loudly as he entered the room.

"Our uncle, Aziel. He died a long time ago. He was Mother's oldest brother," said Tamis.

"And he was called 'Adzil'!" repeated Didi stubbornly.

"Why does it matter so much what exactly he was called?" asked Kim.

"Only because it was on our brother's anklet; on my anklet I have my own name and so does Didi," said Tamis, getting books out. The squabble now ceased; the two boys started their homework with Kim's watchful eye over them.

It was only when on his new bed, unable to sleep, that Kim wondered why Bertis, had an anklet with his uncle's name on it and then, like a niggling pain, he started to wonder why the name "Aziel" had such a ring to it. Eventually he fell asleep and dreamt about trying to find Kelin by a well in a strange town.

He awoke at four-thirty in the morning with a terrible start. Aziel! Of course! It was the name on the anklet that he had taken off the dead man with the horse. How extraordinary! Didi and Tamis's brother, Bertis, wore an anklet with his uncle's name on it ... Why?

"My God!" he almost shouted and sat up in his bed. (Luckily, his new roommate was snoring lightly and didn't awaken.) Kim went over to the window. The view from this side of the house looked out onto some of the great trees in the gardens. He watched as it got lighter and the trees became sharper in outline, until eventually they were all completely visible. His mind was now in a new confusion: was the dead man with the black horse that Kim had buried by the river actually Bertis? Was it possible that he, Kim, was the only person who really knew where Bertis was?

He'd given the diamond and the anklet both to Tiésa for safekeeping and Tiésa had made inquiries about the name on the anklet. Naturally, they both assumed that "Aziel" was the dead man's name. Kim knew for certain that Tiésa had kept the stone because she wanted Kelin to have it if they couldn't find the owner. But the anklet? Had she kept that too? Kim couldn't remember. He remembered Tiésa saying it was very old, but that it had little value. Kim was praying that Tiésa had kept it.

He went down to an early breakfast and asked to speak with Atrell.

"She can speak to no-one today. She's not well," said her maid.

"Oh! But it's urgent!" Kim exclaimed, in spite of himself.

"She's expressly asked not to be disturbed." And the maid closed the door.

With Camdovin away and until now the failure of his searches, Atrell had become more and more sombre, weaker, less able to cope with the day to day running of Ardair. Of course, with or without Atrell, the household ran smoothly, with the two boys diligent in their support of her. But the inhabitants of the house were more subdued: they all went about in a mist of uncertainty and waiting.

Kim's mind was racing. I suppose the fact that Camdovin is away, as well as the gruelling nature of the search, makes it more agonising, he thought, wondering whether there was someone else he could speak to.

In the next moment, Kim was running down the stairs in a bid to find Jisha and ask her an urgent question. He found her in the scullery, dealing with the remains of breakfast and arranged to meet her outside, in the garden, near to the fruit and vegetables where there was a table and chairs for the servants' break-time.

Ten minutes later, Jisha was with him.

"I've only got a minute as I have to prepare lunch,"

she said anxiously.

"Well, it's this," Kim said. "I have a problem with a friend. I won't go into details." He was fudging here, as he really was not able to go into details. "But the customs where I am from, in Grailand are so different, and I need to know what they are here."

"Customs for what?" Jisha asked.

"Well, when a person dies. Does it matter how long it takes to bury them?"

"Oh. I see! Burying people …" She looked worried. "In Memarn? Customs here in Memarn …" she said. "Well here, if a person dies, they must be buried within two days. Yes …two days," she repeated, almost to herself.

"Is that whatever the cause of death is?" asked Kim.

"Yes. As far as I know, whatever the cause of death, burial has to be within two days."

"And what if they die in great pain?" persisted Kim.

"In great pain? Well, it's the same. If in great pain, or under torture, or something like that, then a special prayer has to be said over the body, as far as I know, to release it from its agony."

"Really? A special prayer? Oh, I see."

"Yes. Otherwise their spirit will continue in agony forevermore and can bring shame and agony in turn to the family of the dead person; it can affect very badly the family and children of that family, if that prayer has not been said," Jisha said firmly. "I know that is so. Is it different in Grailand?"

"Yes. It is different there. And I suppose, if it's an

older son, it's worse if there is no prayer."

"Yes. Much worse," said Jisha mournfully, looking over at Kim. "I hope it's not too serious for your friend," she said.

"Well, I hope not. I didn't really understand what he was going on about ..." Kim fibbed again. "I must try and get some time off to help him! Thank you, Jisha, and see you later!" And he rushed off upstairs, to try again to see Atrell. He realised that this must surely be a major part of what Atrell was suffering.

Atrell though was still languishing in her bed, trying to get some sleep. She knew her husband was the best, the kindest and most generous of men; she knew how he had worked his way up to become one of the wealthiest and wisest people in Memarn. As a ten-year-old in her parent's house she had loved him immediately, although of course they did not marry for seven years. Their six children were all deeply loved, and with Bertis being the eldest of them, she knew it would blight the whole family if he were not found either dead or alive. This was the first time she had suffered such anguish.

And now – Kim realised – Atrell and Camdovin were in the same situation as Kim himself. Suddenly each one of them had the key to the other's freedom from generations of pain and hardship. The difference was that Camdovin and Atrell didn't know it yet.

But Atrell was too ill to see anyone today. Kim pleaded with Gralun. "Please, Master Gralun, this is a truly urgent matter!"

"She cannot be seen and that's that!" Gralun told him.

"But what I've got to discuss with her relates to what is making her so ill! I need to know one thing only ..."

"*You* need to know!" boomed Gralun. He was annoyed that this boy, who had come from nowhere a few months ago, had wormed his way into an intimacy with the master and now with the mistress.

"What is so important to you that can affect the mistress's suffering?"

"It's what the boys said yesterday," replied Kim as politely as he could.

"And what may that be?"

"All I can say is that, depending on her answer I might be able to get some important news for her."

"And how might that be?" Gralun, still annoyed, questioned again.

Kim now fell silent and eventually Gralun looked up, saying, "I will ask her once more. I'll tell her it *could* be important for her ..."

"Thank you so much, Master Gralun."

This time it was Gralun who went up to Atrell's quarters to ask permission to send Kim to her, while Kim sat and waited in the anteroom. But again, Gralun was confronted with Atrell's personal maid, Miura.

"It's impossible, Master Gralun. She's sleeping at last. She can't see anyone, however important."

"Kim says it relates to all this, to do with Bertis ..."

"Something to do with Bertis?"

"It's very urgent, he says," Gralun went on.

"Well, I don't know. Has he some news? What is it?"

"He won't tell me. He says he must ask her something

and depending on her answer, he will be able to tell her something about Bertis ... It's confusing!"

"Look, Master Gralun, I can't wake her, not with her having been up all night. It's a blessing she's sleeping! Come back in two hours." With that Miura closed the door and locked it.

Two hours later, now sensing that Kim really had something important to say, Gralun was back again, but Miura's mistress was still asleep. Clearly Gralun had work to do and couldn't spend all his time running up and down the stairs about this – whatever it was!

"Look, Kim, you wait outside Atrell's rooms. Knock on her door in half an hour. I'll get word to the boys that if you're not with them in time, they should get on with their work without you."

After two more knocks, Miura told him the mistress was awake and could see him. He was told to wait in a sitting room where he could see the gardens and, remembering the time he had spent on flower beds and shaped hedges, he watched as one of the new gardeners came into view and looked up at him.

When, eventually, Atrell came in, she made him have a tea with her.

"How are the boys getting on?" she started.

"Well. Very well. It's not about that I am here, ma'am." He was nervous now. She didn't seem aware of the urgency, or that he had been waiting to see her since early morning. "I need to ask you something very important ..."

"What is it, Kim?" She was surprised by his tone.

"It's about the search for Bertis. – I mean, I may know something."

"About Bertis?" Her face fell.

"The thing is, I may know something very important, but first, well first, I need you to answer me, well, one question. If the answer is "yes" then I have … I must see a trusted friend very … I mean, most urgently!" He was not explaining things properly.

"Yes … If you think you may be able to help with the search …" She faltered.

Kim took a deep breath: "Well the question I have to ask is: does your son Bertis make a habit of wearing an anklet with the name 'Aziel' on it?"

Atrell brought her hands up to her mouth, staring at him in disbelief. Eventually, she let out: "Yes. He does. How could you …?" She stopped and then went on quietly, "Aziel was his uncle, my eldest brother who died ten years ago. Bertis adored him; he took the anklet when Aziel died. He wears it all the time."

"He does? Are you sure?"

"Yes. I'm quite sure. Why? How do you come to know about this?"

"If that is your answer, my lady," Kim answered, ignoring her questions, "I need to request some time off, if you don't mind." Kim was nervous now and a little frightened. This was important. "I may have definite information for you this evening. I'll come back as soon as I can."

"Take the time off, and pray it's good news," she faltered.

"I doubt it'll be *good* news, but it may be better than

not knowing. Can I take one of the donkeys to go into town?"

"Take a horse, for goodness' sake!" she told him.

"Please, ma'am, a donkey is all I need. I cannot take a horse."

"If you wish. But see me as soon as you get back and tell me what this is all about. You know how worried I am."

"Thank you, ma'am," Kim said and ran off, down the stairs and out towards the stables; he knew Etsas would lend him the best donkey there.

Chapter 11
THE SECOND INCARCERATION

By the time Kim arrived at Tiésa's stall in the bazaar, it was after lunch and Tiésa's young assistant, Gedrin, was sitting amongst the herbs. He jumped up when Kim appeared.

"When's Tiésa coming back?" Kim questioned him.

"Not until two-thirty," the boy said.

"Do you know where she is?"

"She's with a patient."

"Could you go and get her? It's urgent. I'll look after the shop."

"I'll try," he said. "I know where she is." And Gedrin ran off while Kim minded the stall, sorting out herbs into containers and waiting for Tiésa. A woman came asking for something to calm her baby's teething and an old man came, pointing to the herb to relieve his aching joints. He watched people come and go through the bazaar and prayed Tiésa hadn't sold the anklet or given it away.

Suddenly, he saw a man coming towards him. It was – what was that soldier's name? Kim couldn't remember; but he sat there, behind the herbalist's stall immobile, with his head bowed, eyes closed, as if asleep, until he opened them very slightly and saw the man was browsing casually through the herbs. He had picked up a bottle of tincture and was reading the label. My God! What would Kim say when the man asked about it? He would recognise him immediately, wouldn't he? And Kim, trapped behind the stall table, had nowhere to run except almost exactly to where the soldier was. A moment later the man turned away as someone questioned him.

"Are you interested in that tincture?" she said to the man. It was Tiésa, arrived just in time.

Kim slid silently off his stool and, trembling, moved slowly to the back area of the stall, the covered alcove, where he knew he could not properly be seen. This was not the moment to be caught by his father's men when he seemed absolutely on the threshold of something so important! He again thanked Kelin silently for the hat and talisman, just about managing to keep him safe.

When at last the man left, Kim was ashen-faced and still shaky.

"Oh, Tiésa!" Where should he start? "Yesterday the boys were arguing about the name their brother, Bertis, had on his anklet."

"Are you alright?" she said, slightly perplexed at the frightened look on his face. "Well, and what was so important about that?"

"Tiésa, the name is 'Aziel'! The same name on the anklet I found on the dead man up near the farm, by the river."

"The dead man. What, the same name .... is it?" She was shocked.

"Have you still got that anklet?" he asked anxiously. "I've been waiting all morning to see Atrell because she's not well and I needed to ask her and then I was praying you hadn't lost it or thrown it away because you said it had no value and we couldn't find who it belonged to." All this came out in a rush.

"Don't worry. I've still got it," Tiésa said calmly. "I'll get it for you now so that you can show it to Atrell." She moved to the back of the shop, pulling the curtain aside, revealing what looked like more containers with herbs. She rummaged around for a second or two, then returned to Kim.

"Here you are," she said, putting the anklet into Kim's hand.

Kim looked at it. It was not only old, but light and delicate. He turned it over in his hand to reveal the inscription: "Aziel" it said inside the curve of the solid part of the anklet.

"It must be the one," he almost whispered to Tiésa. "I had better take the diamond back as well to show them both to Atrell," Kim said, after a moment.

"I think perhaps you should wait for Camdovin to return. You said you found that diamond in an unusual place, didn't you? A hiding place that you knew of but the bandits did not. Wait for Camdovin before you take it. It will be proof of your honesty. Take only the anklet now …" she said.

"Yes. Good idea."

He then told Tiésa about the man at her stall, and she produced some harmless white powder Kim was to put over his hair, especially the parts that were visible with his hat on.

"That way, a quick look at you will take you for an old man!" She laughed. "Remember, you've got to get back to Ardair. I don't want you being picked up by those men! Ride that donkey back there as if you're asleep on it," she went on. "They'll think you're just an old servant going back to his master, won't they?" And Kim couldn't resist giving her a hug before he left her, his hair powdered with white.

*   *   *

In the kitchen, there was an excited but almost whispered discussion about Kim amongst some of the staff.

"I saw young Kim in the mistress's sitting room this morning – I think it was," said Melmed's nephew, the new under-gardener.

"Did you? I've had my suspicions for a while now," came in Nemesh, who was relishing his superior knowledge in the matter of Kim.

"Well, I heard that Kim claimed to have something very important to do with the search for Bertis and wouldn't say what it was," said another.

"All I thought was that he was waiting all morning to see the mistress."

"I happen to know that Kim has often come back to bed at two in the morning, with piles of books in his arms," Nemesh spoke again. "I once tried, later, to find one of those books, but it wasn't in the library and Damos, whose father has a fruit stall, says he often sees Kim in the bazaar. I think it's very strange the way this young boy has risen from being an under-gardener to tutor to Tamis and Didi in such a short time." All those at the dining table listened, spellbound to Nemesh's ideas and pronouncements. "Not only that," he went on, "but I've found out that he doesn't come from Grailand at all." This was said with flourish and pride.

"Are you sure? How do you know?" asked Gralun, who had come into the room unnoticed and was listening intently. "That is fraud – of a kind," he said. Everyone looked stunned.

"I checked," answered Nemesh. "It was difficult, but I have a friend in one of the government offices there. He was quite certain."

"I heard he may have been in prison," said Jisha timidly, not sure whether she wanted to add to the so-called crimes of this nice boy.

"So maybe he's been stealing the books to sell at the bazaar," said another of the servants.

"And why, only now, does he know something important about the search, when they've been gone almost a month?"

"My God! Who does this boy think he is?" cried Gralun in a fury. "This cannot be tolerated!"

It happened that Kim arrived at the door, back from the bazaar, to overhear the last sentence. He had no idea they were talking about him and was so excited about the anklet that he ran into the room.

There was a shocked hush not only because he had been the subject of so much talk, but also because he seemed to have got flour over parts of his hair! But Kim, intent only on getting the anklet to Atrell as quickly as possible, didn't notice the stares and sidelong glances from around the table, where some of them were still eating.

"Mr Gralun! Please can I talk to you in private?"

"Come, we shall go to my office."

Kim would have gone straight to Atrell but he thought it better that he speak to Gralun first.

"What's it about?" Gralun asked once they were in his room.

"You know what it's about! It's the same as it was this morning, only now I have something concrete for her! It's urgent, Mr Gralun!"

"Urgent in your eyes, it may be. But I'm afraid there have been various stories going around about you, which have only just come to my notice ..." Gralun said, eyeing Kim coldly.

"Stories? What stories?"

"Apparently you have been seen in the mistress's room. On many occasions you have arrived extremely late for bed, carrying a quantity of books which were later thought to be missing from the library. You have also been seen in the bazaar several times ..." This was said very calmly by Gralun as if it were a catalogue of proven crimes, rather than facts with no significance.

"What books are missing?" asked Kim.

"I don't know any titles. All I know is that one person

tried to find a book he had seen you with earlier and found it not in the library ..."

"That's because it was either in the study room, or one of the boys had it! It's complete rubbish!" his voice was raised.

"Another thing we've discovered is that you are not from Grailand. ..."

"Who said this?" Kim clenched his fists in a fury. He was starting to tremble with fear: he *had* lied to them about Grailand.

"We have had a discussion about this and have come to a decision," Gralun said mysteriously, without answering his question.

"What do you mean ...?"

"The master will deal with you when he gets back."

"Deal with what? You don't even know!"

"That's just it. We don't even know what it is you're on about!" Gralun sounded angry now. "No-one knows. Even the mistress, who you absolutely had to see earlier on today. When we asked her, she didn't know exactly what you wanted to show her. She thought it could be good news, but she wasn't sure. The fact is, Kim, we know very little about you. You seem to spend large amounts of time in the mistress's quarters or in the library."

"Large amounts of time in the library, yes!" He was shouting now in desperation. "Reading or studying! I've only been to the mistress's quarters twice. Once because she asked me to come there, with a maid there while we talked. The second time was today. We talk about the boys. That's part of my job!"

"But you came here as a gardener!"

"Yes, I came as a gardener. What's wrong with that?"

"And what are you really? Gardener or tutor?" Gralun glowered at him.

Kim suddenly clammed up. He couldn't cope with this. The questions didn't make sense. Eventually he said as quietly as he could: "Please, Mr Gralun, be good enough to tell the mistress that I have something concrete …" He stopped for a moment, unsure of how to go on. Then continued: "I have something that I believe belongs to Bertis which I want to show to her and only to her. It's a delicate matter." Kim realised he would have to explain how he'd got hold of the anklet. Gralun wasn't the person to tell all this. It would have to be Atrell – or, even better, Camdovin.

"Oh, no you will not, my young man!" said Gralun, firmly. He got up to bar his way, then shouted: "Guards!" At that moment, two big men appeared who now stood either side of Kim.

"You're confined to a special room until such a time as Camdovin or one of his advisers can decide about you. The master will be back within the week."

"I don't understand what I have done!" Kim cried out.

"There have been some discoveries made which we think will be interesting to the master. You said you came from Grailand but were forced to come here in search of work." Gralun paused, looking at him. "But there is no record of you having come from Grailand, nor that any of the schools there play all the sports that you have done here. Now you say you have something belonging to Bertis. This puts you under further suspicion. It is difficult to believe anything you say, amongst all your lies. It may have some connection with Bertis's disappearance, but that could be a lie too."

"It does have to do with Bertis." Kim's breathing had become tight and panicked. "That's why I need to talk with the mistress. I beg you to let her hear me. Those other things I can explain." He was desperate. "I can and will explain everything to Atrell or Camdovin!" he repeated, but Gralun only shrugged; and the trouble was that Kim knew they had reason to be suspicious of him: he was not the person he pretended to be. Now he was escorted by the two guards down to a small chamber where he was given soup and bread and locked in. After pacing in a fury for an hour, he eventually managed to calm down, comforting himself with the thought that the master would soon be back. That was the only piece of good news. Perhaps Camdovin would listen to him.

*　*　*

Only Camdovin didn't return until after a week because another lead came up, which he felt compelled to follow. And a lead could take you all over the place. So, for the next ten days Kim languished in his new prison. This one had comforts and was clean; he was given proper food as well as the company of one or other of the guards. His friends in the household were too shocked or frightened to come and see him in case they should be tainted with being traitorous. Even Didi and Tamis were forbidden to see him. They allowed him books, but no pen and paper in case he started "inventing stories about himself again", they said.

He prayed that when Camdovin got back he would listen to him.

Kim was due to be severely tried yet again, because when eventually Camdovin did get back, naturally the master's main concern was the health of his wife and children. On top of that, as often happens to powerful men, he was told all sorts of stories about Kim, few of which were actually true. Also, he was overtired and desperately worried about his son, missing and presumed dead; the household was in an uproar, with his wife and children in a state of despair, as well as Kim confined to the one room.

Camdovin had difficulty understanding what had happened. Gralun tried to explain: "The thing is, it's possible he has been stealing books to sell at the market, but crucially, Nemesh, who knows him well, has made inquiries in Grailand and found that he is definitely not from there."

"But he told me he came from there, was educated there …" Camdovin was at a loss.

"He told all of us. Something he said made Nemesh suspicious."

"I found him a very engaging boy. And clever. A wonderful sportsman. He really could teach those boys of mine. How odd. Everything is so upside down, I don't know what to think. Tamis and Didi love him. And yet he is a fraudster!"

"He seems to have come here under false pretences. We don't know why. Books maybe? And now he is claiming to know something about Bertis."

"He says he knows something about Bertis? Well, that could be another lie." Camdovin wiped his brow and looked at Gralun wearily. "Maybe his purpose was to lure me into some business scheme … I'll have to find out. I'll talk to him tomorrow, when I have rested." And Camdovin moved off with a heavy heart, fearful of what he might find out the next day.

* * *

Ideas and conjectures about Kim were endless and Camdovin, miserable and dejected, listened to all of these. His instinct was to dismiss him immediately, without further ado, but Atrell, who had done nothing about Kim's imprisonment for fear of creating further difficulties, now pleaded with her husband.

"Listen to what Kim has to say, because I really believe he may know something important!"

"Do you think he's to be trusted?"

"Well, our children trusted him for a long time. Our two youngest boys aren't stupid …"

"That's true. And, in fact, I trusted him. It's all these stories that make me doubt him." He paused for a moment, then said, "Alright. I'll see him." And, after resolving to steel himself against the obvious charms and cleverness of this very young man, Camdovin went down to see him.

During his time in the cell under Ardair, Kim had not once been searched, which meant that he had still managed to hide both the talisman and the anklet. He had also devised a way of extracting the anklet without having to undo the waistband at all, while keeping hidden the priceless talisman which he still believed would in the end keep him safe.

As Kim sat reading, exactly two weeks after he had been brought down here, he heard a familiar voice. It was Camdovin, and he all but rushed towards his master in joy. But he stopped himself, especially on seeing the look of distaste on Camdovin's face. Kim's first idea had been to tell Camdovin everything immediately in total honesty. Now, seeing that things were going to be difficult even with his adored master, he realised that he would have to go slowly and carefully and that he should be mindful of how he told Camdovin the full story.

He made a deep bow to Camdovin and then looked at him squarely.

"I hear you have deceived me …" Camdovin boomed at him with his inimitable voice.

"I own, Master, that I did. But I had good reason."

"How can a person have a good reason to deceive?"

"'Deceive', Master, is too strong a word. It implies harm. I have done you no harm. What I have done is to pretend to be someone I am not. For a purpose, but not to harm you, I promise. Have you found any harm?"

Here Camdovin muttered something about stealing

186

books and lying about his origins and general falseness.

"Sometimes, sir, a person might have reasons to pursue something and somewhat change his identity to be able to forward those pursuits."

At this, Camdovin eyed Kim brightly, in recognition of his own change of name all those years ago, unaware of course that Kim knew about that.

"I am told quite a few things about you," he said. "One is that Nemesh discovered you have lied about where you came from and your reasons for being here. Two, he also says that you've been stealing books from the library and selling them, though no-one can find which books are missing; three, one of the kitchen staff thinks you may have been in prison; four, Gralun says you claim to have news about my lost son; and five, since I have asked everyone what they know about you, Didi says that you are not only a wizard at sports, but also a wizard with horses and yet you claim only ever to ride a donkey."

"What can I say, Master? There is only one of those things that is not true."

"And that is …?"

"I have never stolen a book in my life."

"So, you lied about all the other things! You must explain yourself," Camdovin responded.

"I can, and will, of course, explain myself, Master. But – if I may – I will start with my information about your son, because that is by far the most urgent. Also, when you know what it is, you might have more sympathy with the other reason I am here." With that, Kim took from his waistband the anklet that had belonged to the dead man by the river. "This," he said, "is what I wanted to show the mistress, so that she could confirm it's the one worn by Bertis." He handed it to Camdovin. "It has inscribed on it the name '*Aziel*'."

Camdovin took the anklet gently in his hand.

"My God. Yes. My wife's brother's name. How do you have it?" Camdovin held the anklet, inspecting it, with its patterned border and its ornate script "*Aziel*". After a moment he said: "I'm almost sure it is. My wife will know," he said. "I'll take it to her!" And he left abruptly with the anklet.

Ten minutes later he was back with Atrell. They both sat down, Camdovin directly in front of Kim. Looking him in the eye, he said, "How do you come to have this?"

"I want to tell you ... but ..." This was going to be difficult for Kim. "But there are some things I must beg you not to question for the time being. I will answer all the questions later. But the first thing is to deal with the question of your son, who, I must tell you, I believe to be dead and buried for about five months." He said this with care, watching Atrell to make sure she didn't take it too badly, knowing also that the fact of his burial would be a relief to them both.

"Oh, no ..." Atrell's hands went to her mouth as her face creased in pain.

Camdovin heaved a melancholy sigh, but then questioned, "How do you know this? How can you be sure?"

"I buried him myself," Kim said simply and proceeded

to tell them about his descent down the mountain, of finding the anklet under the boot, and the diamond sewn into the waistband. "It is a thing we do in my family; we sew jewels into the waistband. People don't look there. It was automatic for me to make sure. I buried him by the river and then went on to sell my maize."

Camdovin looked at Atrell for a moment and nodded. "And can you take me there?"

"Of course, Master, if I can ride on a donkey ..."

"Ride a donkey? You'll ride a horse!"

"No, Master, I have to ride a donkey."

"So be it," said Camdovin wearily. All he wanted now was to be able to bury the body of his son in the vault here, in the grounds. "And what became of the diamond?" Camdovin asked.

"The diamond I can get for you, as soon as I am freed from this prison!"

"And how do I know that you weren't the one who killed my son to steal all the other jewels? You admit you've been in prison ..."

"Because, Master, why would I do such a thing? I had bags of maize to sell and I was going to Trasimid. I am not a murderer or thief. I myself was left for dead by bandits on the other side of that very same mountain and was later wrongly imprisoned."

"But there's something you haven't told me!" exclaimed Camdovin.

"What's that?"

"You can't be telling the truth!" he cried. "You must be a thief!"

"No …! What have I stolen?"

"The horse! Where's the horse? This must all be a pack of lies! I don't know how you came by this anklet but you'd tell me about the horse if you were telling the truth!"

"I can tell you about the horse, Master!" Kim was shaken now. Why wouldn't Camdovin believe him?

"Tell me where that horse is now and I will believe what you say. Such a horse would never be captured. He was so clever he would run for days before being taken from the man who nurtured him from birth! What colour was the horse?" Camdovin asked suddenly.

"The horse I saw was absolutely black."

"Where is he now?"

"I might even be able to get him back if you are very fond of him, though I think it may cost something. I'll show you where he is, just as I will take you to where Bertis is buried and I'll give you back your diamond. After all that, if you then believe me, I'll tell you why I came here in the first place and why I told some lies."

"Very well," said Camdovin looking at his wife for her agreement, which she gave. "You can have a room upstairs. We leave tomorrow, I think." He turned to her again and she nodded. "But you will be guarded and have food brought to you."

"I understand, sir."

As they left, Camdovin told the guards to take Kim to the second floor.

"One of you guard him at all times. Feed him properly and give him some exercise. I want him fit for our journey to the Binon Mountains."

Chapter 12
THE TRAVELLING PARTY

By noon the next day the small convoy was ready. The cart, which held a coffin and some tents as well as food for the journey, was drawn by two horses. They took a donkey for Kim, although he would mainly sit in the cart, and there were four men on horseback including a priest, together with Atrell, who insisted on coming, and of course Camdovin. The idea was that this sad and grieving party would take just under a week to get to the foothills of the Binon Mountains.

First, they had to see Tiésa at the bazaar and when they arrived it was Gedrin minding the stall again.

He rushed off to get her and after ten minutes he was back with Tiésa.

After looking around to check that there were none of his father's men nearby, Kim turned to Camdovin. "This is Tiésa, a great friend of the man who saved my life in the Binon Mountains, after I was attacked by bandits."

"Camdovin. I am pleased to meet you." Camdovin shook her hand seriously. "I believe you have something of ours …"

"The diamond. I gave it to you to look after," Kim prompted.

"Of course. I have it." And she went into the cubby hole behind her stall. A moment later she was back with the stone, which she handed to Camdovin.

"Yes," said Camdovin, "it's the one I gave him to hide and only to use in case of dire need." With that, as if he had been doing it all his life, Camdovin placed the diamond into the lining of his waistband and, with two threads, fastened it securely inside. Kim gasped at the speed with which he did this.

"A useful trick!" Camdovin said to Tiésa. "I am showing you because I trust you, old woman. And," he looked at Kim, "you, I am beginning to trust."

"I thought it was my family who had invented this method of outwitting robbers!" Kim blurted out. Camdovin looked surprised but said nothing. As they were leaving Camdovin turned to Tiésa.

"If you need anything, you know where my house is."

"Thank you, kind sir," answered Tiésa. "But Kim is the one by far in greatest need of your assistance."

Camdovin, still in ignorance of Kim's real purpose here, turned to him and said, "If what you say is all true, I promise you will be freed."

* * *

Now the party moved on, resting at inns or camping in the fields in the warm, late summer evenings. They reached the foothills and came near to the village where the horse had been part-sold and put to work. Kim didn't tell Camdovin where the horse was yet, but watched carefully as they went past the field where the farmers had taken the horse to see if it was still there. No horse of any kind was visible, only people working in a field. Perhaps it was behind the clump of trees, Kim comforted himself. Perhaps it was being kept in the stable. Or, he worried, perhaps the horse had been taken somewhere far away.

The party moved on, searching for a place for the night, past the farm, up the winding mountain road, less of a road here and more of a path, up towards the narrowing River Wisees, which tumbled down the mountainside.

The next day they continued uphill, with Kim on alert, looking towards the river to see the place where he thought he had buried Bertis.

As the afternoon came, Kim gave a yell, calling out for them to stop. He jumped off the cart and walked through the trees as Camdovin quickly dismounted and followed him.

The trees were not thick here, but there were clearings like this one all along the edge of the river and the grass, as ever, was high and thick and green.

"It was somewhere here, I think," Kim called over to Camdovin, moving backwards, down the hill amongst the trees. "I buried him at right-angles to the river. I had nothing to dig with so I just laid everything I could find on top of him, mainly these thick clods of grass, including parts of the overhanging bank ... But it doesn't overhang here. Perhaps it's a bit further up."

Kim and Camdovin moved uphill again, keeping to the bank, and at last they came to a grassy mound.

"Here, I think this is it!"

The mound was easy to miss as it had been taken over by grass and greenery near the river.

"This is definitely it," Kim said again. "I remember it was in line on two sides with nearby trees." He pointed. Two glistening birch trees stood nearby, one in line with the head of the mound, the other to the right of it. Camdovin went to get the others, and the men came with shovels and pickaxes, while Atrell carried a wide, deep cloth, for wrapping up the body. It took them twenty minutes to uncover the badly decomposed body and another quarter of an hour to get it into the thick shroud laden with eucalyptus leaves. All the while, Camdovin was urging them,

"Take care, now, slowly ..." with Atrell at his side, weeping silently. Atrell had started off helping to uncover the body, but when they came to a piece of his clothing, she ran away in pain. Camdovin went after her.

"Remember, this is for the best, my dear. We will be able to give him a proper burial and say the prayer over him. Please. Let's do it together."

Eventually, when the body was completely uncovered, Atrell turned back to them, gave a quick look at what was hardly a corpse any longer to make sure, all the same, that it was her son, then covered him from head to toe with the thick, pungent cloth. She tucked in the short end of the great shroud and with the help of the others rolled the remains of her son up, out of his resting place and into the shroud. The ends were then tucked in and lovingly sewn up by his mother and the men carried him to the cart. There he was placed into the coffin, which was also heavily laden with eucalyptus leaves. They all stood there for a moment, as the priest gave his blessing, and then quietly moved off to mount their horses, as Camdovin came towards Kim and embraced him.

"Thank you, my boy. I will never be able to thank you enough." And Kim looked at him with tears in his eyes, Kim himself thanking whichever power it was that had enabled him to bury this poor young man in the only way that he could.

As Camdovin walked heavily back to his horse, Kim got back into the cart next to the coffin.

"Now," he called loudly out to Camdovin and the others, "we go back the same way, to see if we can find the horse!"

So, the little convoy turned around and, with its sad trophy, moved downwards again. Camdovin wondered what could have happened to Lundell, Bertis's aide, who had not been heard of for all this time and who had probably also been killed and thrown into the river.

When they reached the village, the light was fading. Kim got off his cart and went over to Camdovin and Atrell in the front of the caravanserai.

"Could we all wait here a moment, while I ask the farmer if we can stay in his field …?" Kim asked.

"Of course, young man. Whatever you wish." Camdovin, despite mourning his son, looked at Kim with admiration and fondness. Kim then disappeared down the path towards the farm.

When he came back, he had the farmer with him.

"The farmer says we can camp in his field and he will sell us eggs and milk and provide us with water."

Camdovin thanked the farmer and the party, with their precious cargo, now moved along the path towards the farm and from there to the field. Meanwhile, Kim said quietly to Camdovin, "The farmer would like to show you something ..." And, in the twilight, the farmer led man and boy down another pathway, through a clump of trees and into another field where there were three horses. "What was the name of Bertis's horse, sir?"

"'Celendiss', he was called," answered Camdovin.

"Try calling him, see what happens ..." Kim said gently.

So Camdovin called Celendiss in the way that he had always done since the horse was born, and of course the black horse came trotting up to him immediately, nuzzling Camdovin and being fondled by his old master.

"He's sired a son, sir," said the farmer. "We've been ever so happy with him."

Then Kim turned to Camdovin. "He's a wonderful horse. So intelligent. You know, he watched me carefully while I searched your dear son, and while I buried him. I didn't dare make a wrong move because your horse was guarding him and watching me like a hawk! Then, after my donkey and I had gone quite a way down the hill towards this farm, we heard an echoing clip-clop sound which went on and on. Eventually I saw this beautiful horse coming down the mountainside after us. He kept his distance, you know. Just following. We had to entice him with oats to get him to come into the farm. They paid me some extra for the maize I'd brought because of the black horse."

Camdovin laughed again with the thought of being with his bright horse once more.

"Now it's just a question of whether the farmer will let him go ..." Kim said quietly.

"Tell me," Camdovin went over to the farmer, followed closely by Celendiss, "what do you think he's worth now?"

"He's been invaluable to us, sir. Works hard and I've never come across a horse as clever as him. We've called him Burla. We think the mare's pregnant again, so that'll be two foals he's given us." The farmer watched as the horse and master nuzzled each other like long lost friends. "He's certainly fond of you, sir."

"He's known me since he was born. He was my son's horse. They grew up together. The fastest, cleverest horse we've ever come across, aren't you?" The horse nuzzled him again.

"I wonder how he escaped the bandits ..." Kim murmured.

"Speed. He's so fast," said Camdovin. "How long had Bertis been dead, do you think? About two days, wasn't it?"

"A day or so. I was filling my water bottle, and then this beautiful horse led me to the body."

"We thought my son's companion, Lundell, was probably thrown into the river ..." Camdovin was addressing the farmer again. "Did you hear of any other deaths here around six months ago?"

"I'm sorry, I heard about your great sadness, sir. Let me think. There was a body found in the river down the hillside around that time. They found it in Idena, half way to Trasimid. Don't know who it was, though."

It was getting dark now and the three of them walked back towards the farm and beyond, where Atrell and the others were preparing some food.

"How much do you want for the black horse?" asked Camdovin.

"Oh, dear sir!" cried the farmer. "I can see how he loves you ... The trouble is, we need two working horses for the farm ..."

"How would it be if I gave you enough for two more working horses, with the first option on both the foals at a later stage?" Camdovin had taken out some notes of a large denomination and was counting out twenty of them. "Two thousand crowns would be enough, wouldn't it?"

"Too much, sir, far too much! I don't know ... She'll be sad without him. The mare. She'll be very sad."

"Well ... What if we were to bring him here for three months every year for the next five years. That way she can have his company for a bit and she may have another foal," said Camdovin, delighted with his idea and with the prospect of having Bertis's beloved stallion back again.

"Yes, sir! I'll agree to that!" The farmer laughed.

"Celendiss will pull my son's coffin at the funeral," Camdovin said quietly, as he and Kim walked back towards the tents that had been erected in the field.

On their way down towards Trasimid, passing Idena, they dropped one of the men off at the village to learn what he could about the body found in the river and see if it was that of Lundell.

But Kim's job was still to be done. He knew that the time had come when Camdovin would not be able to reject his difficult request; Kim would, after all this time, get some answers to the questions that had been plaguing him.

Chapter 13
MOMENT OF TRUTH

When, four days and nights later, they arrived back at the big house, arrangements were immediately made for a funeral in a few days. This was held with great pomp and ceremony as the black horse Celendiss pulled the coffin through the grounds, to the vault which had been built some time ago with Bertis's parents in mind. During the ceremony attended by family, friends and staff, Camdovin spoke about his son, Bertis, in glowing and loving terms. Then he went on: "I would like to add to this that if it hadn't been for the kindness, generosity and I have to say courage of my friend here, Kim, we might never have known of Bertis's fate or been able to bring his body to our family vault for a fitting burial – nor indeed would we have had Bertis's adored horse, Celendiss, to pull the coffin. Kim knew nothing of our family at that time, but simply did the humane action of burying a person, saving his soul in this way. Kim has my undying gratitude for, in some way, righting the terrible wrong that was done to Bertis."

Despite the kind words of Camdovin about Kim at the funeral, the next day there was talk in the kitchens about Kim's suitability as tutor to Camdovin's youngest sons, stoked up in the main by Nemesh's insistence that Kim was a liar.

"I mean, why did he pretend to come from Grailand?" asked Nemesh, back on his bandwagon.

"And why did he bury a complete stranger who had been murdered?" went on one of the under-cooks. "Maybe he was looking for more plunder."

"Maybe he was the one who murdered him!" exclaimed another young man peeling potatoes. "He's a known liar. Maybe he's also a murderer."

Nemesh smiled, knowing that was unlikely, but enjoying the way the conversation was going. After all, it wasn't just him. Jisha was adamant that Kim had said he had been in prison.

One of the men, Erun, who had guarded Kim when he had been locked in the downstairs room, heard these persistent rumours and intrigues and, having become good friends with Kim since the young prince's imprisonment, now told Kim about the gossip.

"I think you'd better go and explain yourself to the master quickly, before he hears of these things again."

"He's asked me to come and see him anyway. I'm a bit nervous about it, I've got so much to say … and to ask." He hesitated. This was the moment he'd been waiting for and yet he was terrified. He turned again to Erun. "I'll try and see him now! Could you warn the boys that I'll be late for their studies?"

Erun agreed and Kim rushed off to Camdovin's study. When he got there, his heart was in his mouth, but the answer to his knock on the door was a friendly, "Come in!" And seeing who it was, sitting at his desk, Camdovin forestalled him: "You have come to tell me about the stories you made up ... Come, sit down."

Kim sat down in a chair opposite Camdovin and blurted out: "They were stories I made up so that I could have work in your house!" This did not come out at all as Kim had planned. "Master," Kim went on, "I had a very important reason for wishing to know you."

There was a hesitation, a momentary fear in Camdovin's eyes even, as he weighed up what it was Kim was about to tell him.

"A reason to get to know me?" This was the last thing that Camdovin had expected or wanted. Again, for a moment he wondered if this was friend or foe. "What reason?" he said eventually.

"I come from a family where terrible things have happened ..."

"I see ..." Camdovin looked worried.

"These things ... I do not know what they are. Only that on her deathbed, my mother said I must find out so that I could right the wrongs and prevent each further generation from suffering an uncontrollable and terrible curse, an anguish which could go on from one generation to the next until the end of time."

Camdovin now looked pale. His face showed a fear that Kim could never have imagined, staring at Kim in disbelief.

At last, Camdovin said quietly, "And how can I help you with this ... this kind of torture of the mind?"

"You, my dear master," and here Kim was torn with what he *had* to ask him and the wish to protect this admired man from further pain, "you are the only one who knows what these terrible things are; the only person who can set my mind at rest and enable the future generations of my family to live in peace." He stopped, put his head in his hands, then looked up at Camdovin.

"I?" Camdovin hesitated again. "And who are your family?" he almost whispered. But it was clear from Camdovin's face that he already knew.

Kim now took from the top of his waistband the diamond that his mother had given him. He put the gem down in front of Camdovin.

"I am Prince Kim of Strela. My father is King Demble, of the House of Koremine, and my mother was Queen Donata. When my mother was dying, she gave me this to give to you."

Camdovin was staring with disbelief at the stone, now in his hand. Then he nodded slowly. Kim went on: "She said she gave you another one exactly the same and that you would recognise it. She told me that only one man, named Balquin, knew the truth about the terrible quarrel that killed my grandmother, Queen Porla, that this man not only knew what was said, unlike anyone else except those in the room, but that he also possessed papers to prove what he knew. This is what she told me."

Still holding the diamond, Camdovin now got up from his chair and turned away from Kim. He was obviously in some shock as he went to his great window, staring out in disbelief. For a moment he turned back to look at the young prince waiting anxiously at the other side of his desk. Eventually he came back to his chair, facing Kim.

"I am very sad to hear of Donata's death. She was a good person … But why didn't you show me this diamond before?"

"I wanted to on several occasions, but it seemed inappropriate. I didn't think you'd have any reason to believe me. Later, I just thought you'd accuse me of stealing it from you, since my mother said yours is exactly the same!"

"I sold mine long ago," said Camdovin simply. "But I recognise this." He turned away again, closing his eyes in thought. After a few moments, with Kim still watching in suspense, Camdovin turned back towards him with a great sigh.

"It's true, I used to be called Balquin. I did everything to overcome what I learned that night and an essential part of it was to change my name … But … I'm so sorry about your mother," he said again. "You are like her, aren't you? I think that's what affected me when I first saw you … Yes, I worked at Koremine Castle when that argument took place – screaming battle, more like. We were all frightened by the shouting and desperate to know what it was all about. So, I went up." He said this shaking his head, as if it were the worst thing he could ever have done.

Kim waited for him to continue.

"I went up those long winding stairs and when I got to the top, I crept along the narrow corridor. The sound was more frightening the nearer you got. It echoed everywhere. At last, I got to the cubby hole and hid behind the canopy. I was so relieved to be safe that I took a while to recover – and all because of a promised kiss from the lovely Sela – which I never got!" He gave a short laugh. "I wrote down what I heard while it was still fresh in my mind."

"Is that the document my mother talked of?"

"No, I don't think so. No, the document is something else; legal proof of what happened. That document is in the hands of lawyers or accountants of King Ambab, in Beran, proving illegal dealings which led to a mass poisoning and contamination of people in Strela. A company called Kardra and Co. ... I think King Ambab, who is a good king, was given only some of the details and didn't know the full picture; but I believe he still owns those documents." He paused. "No, what *I* wrote down was what I heard: the quarrel itself, the first I heard of the poisonings; the crime which caused the curse. When a bad deed happens, it doesn't simply happen on its own, unconnected to the rest of life. It affects all and everything around it. In effect, creating a curse, especially on people who are innocently linked to the bad deed. However simple the bad deed is, the repercussions can be terrible and all permeating."

After a moment Kim ventured, "Would I be allowed to read that document?" He looked at Camdovin with anxious expectancy.

"I'm sure," responded Camdovin sadly, "that what I wrote is of interest, but it is all far away, in a place I went to after your mother saved my life."

"My mother?"

"Yes, Donata as she was then. At the time she was betrothed to your father. Although she got to know about the notes I had made, she never actually read them herself. She said it wouldn't affect the betrothal." He paused again, then went on: "No, that night, after I'd heard all the screaming, I came back to the kitchens in a terrible state and I didn't sleep for days. When Queen Porla was found dead in her room, I decided it was time to go."

"Do you know how she died?"

"It was a mystery and I was frightened someone could find out I'd heard the quarrel; I felt in danger myself. I left a couple of days after she died. At first, I had no thought of writing down what I'd heard."

"But you did, didn't you?"

"I did. These events – the words that had been said – were swirling around in my head; I felt completely battered by it all. So, I decided to write it all down, word for word." Camdovin sat at his desk imitating the way he had written those notes, all that time ago: slowly, painstakingly following the line of each letter.

"It took me about three days, but it calmed me. I went on towards Beran, but I'd run out of food and, as I got to the Klandin Mountains – still hiding because I was terrified the king's men were out to find me – it got much colder. There were no animals to catch, snow was falling and I was weak. After some days, I heard people coming, so I jumped into a ditch to hide, but I twisted my ankle and they heard me yell in pain. They found me and took me to your mother's house in the valley. She nursed me until I was well and I told her something of what had happened.

"She was already betrothed to your father, when I asked her if she would hand me over to King Strearn, her future father in law. She said it wasn't her business and, as I seemed honest, she would say nothing. You must remember I was only eighteen. She was about six years older. I think she knew something of what Prince Demble was like, only her parents wanted her to marry him and perhaps she thought she could change him for the better.

"Eventually I told her why I was so scared. I didn't say *what* I'd heard, only that I'd heard a terrible row. I also told her I'd written down what was said, so if someone ever needed to know the awfulness of that quarrel, they could read it. She was not interested in reading it herself, which was a great relief, as I was afraid she would tell Prince Demble about me.

"When I left your mother's house, she promised not to talk about me unless it were a matter of life and death. And she gave me the diamond in case of need. Although I loved and trusted her, I could never be sure she wouldn't be forced to tell my secret. That's why I changed my name. I always thought that if anyone really needed to find me, they would find a way to do so."

"And what did you do then?" asked Kim.

"I went on to Beran, where King Ambab rules, and where I've heard now his daughter Princess Sagesse is very ill. I worked at the palace, helping with the horses.

I wanted to find out if King Ambab knew of what I'd heard; how guilty he was. I discovered that he was generally kind and loved."

"My father and King Ambab don't get on anymore," said Kim.

"At the time, they had been friends. And although I was only a stable boy, I kept fearing your grandfather would issue an edict against me, proclaiming me a traitor, so I kept myself to myself.

"When I left Koremine Castle I was terrified, and when, eventually, I came to Memarn, I was still frightened that someone would drag me back to your grandfather. My wealth came to me quite unexpectedly. Then I went south, to Karmassos. I didn't stay long. Just long enough to buy a new set of clothes, four horses and hire a manservant, my old friend Etsas. Anyway, I came back with a new name. And so you see me now, known in Trasimid and all of Memarn as Camdovin."

"But how did you make so much money?" Kim asked, in awe.

Camdovin got up from his desk and started moving round the room. "It was luck to start with. Once you have a bit, it is easy to go on making more – if you are self-disciplined. It's getting out of poverty that's the most difficult. And I had sold your mother's diamond long before this.

"At the time, I was working for a blacksmith, Plosit, and I lived in a hovel just over the hill, where there was a bit of green grass. Often, the rich men didn't come for their horses on the day they'd been newly shod, and

Plosit used to get me to take those horses up by my hovel for the night, on the patch of green. Usually, after a day or two a servant would come to collect the horse. Well in this case, the owner didn't come. I found out he had died suddenly and the household was in uproar. I kept bringing the beast in, but no-one came. After about a month I stopped bringing her in, just kept her tethered by my shack. I realised no-one was coming for her and that if I played my cards right, I could be richer by a valuable horse.

"I told Plosit that the owner had come while he was out. He always made owners pay as soon as they arrived, so he didn't lose any money. Anyway, he believed me and I reasoned to myself that Plosit was not being harmed. The next day I told him I'd received word that my father was ill in Strela and I'd have to leave."

"And you changed your name after you left Plosit?"

"Yes, dear old Plosit. Is that how you found me?"

"Yes. He gave my friend Tiésa some contacts, which led to you. Difficult, though!"

Camdovin laughed: "It needed someone determined."

"How did you get to where you are now?"

"As soon as I acquired a bit of money, I bought clothes to change my image. Then I got my manservant, Etsas, and so on. I felt safe and much freer with my new name. I didn't have to look over my shoulder. I built up my trading company and from there I specialised in building works and now I do both the building and some trading."

"I see ... It's amazing ..." Kim said, in wonder. "And you're sure the documents proving what you heard are at King Ambab's court, aren't you?"

"I *believe* some legal papers relating to some of the things were kept by King Ambab or his accountants. But I've never seen them. I am almost certain the king had no understanding of their importance. I wrote the notes for my own peace of mind – a 'report' if you want, which I hid in the grounds of the palace."

"Vocimere Palace?" Kim asked, surprised.

"Vocimere Palace. Yes."

"Whereabouts did you hide these papers, then?" asked Kim quickly.

Since Camdovin had mentioned Sagesse's illness, Kim was now desperate to learn the truth: about his grandmother's death; about what had happened; about the curse and its power – not only on his family. Also, he felt sure that, just as King Ambab was maybe unwittingly involved, so was Sagesse's illness caused by this curse. He was also starting to recognise that his own almost uncontrollable fury at times was caused by the curse, just as was his grandmother's death. But what else could it have caused, or was being affected now?

"I'll tell you where these notes are hidden, but on one condition," said Camdovin eyeing Kim carefully.

"What is that?"

"On condition that you not only read the notes and study them, but that you also act on them. In other words, you must get from King Ambab the relevant documents so that you can confront your father."

"Oh, I intend to do that!" said Kim decisively. "I will do everything in my power to get rid of this curse. It is destroying – has destroyed – people I love!"

Camdovin looked at Kim with deep approval. "If you can do that, then the secret that has devastated so many lives, not only in your family, but in many other families, will then have no further power; it will be like a spell that has been broken. When a nasty secret is out, it stops doing harm. The living will all be able to pursue the lives they want and flourish. That is all. That's enough, isn't it?" Camdovin added.

"Yes. If I can do it!"

"If you can do it, of course. But I think you've done quite a lot already, haven't you? Difficult things … as well as saving my family!" He was smiling.

"Whereabouts did you hide those notes?"

"In the grounds of the palace, towards the east side, amongst the trees there's a very old oak tree, all hollow and musty. Inside, there is just enough room for a man and there's a broken root there that makes a kind of bench. Well, at about two metres high, above the entrance to the hollow, there's a much smaller ledge. On that is a roll of paper wrapped in leather. These are the notes."

"I know that oak," Kim said to Camdovin, softly. "I used to play in it as a child …"

There was a long pause as they each thought about the hollowed oak tree and what it meant to them, separately. Then Kim went on: "There's another thing that is worrying me, and that is that I have noticed my father's men around here, in Trasimid. I can only think that he may have found out that I am searching for you and is trying to stop me."

"That is possible … You must take care!" Camdovin looked alarmed, turning to face Kim. "Have they seen you come to this house?"

"No. I don't think so."

"I did hear that the king, your grandfather, found out about me having overheard the quarrel and sent men out to search for me. I'll never know where they looked, but luckily they never found me. That's why I was so frightened; that's why I had to change my name."

"Maybe my father has found out somehow or realised that my mother sent me to look for you. The man in the mountain who saved my life gave me some old clothes to wear, including a hat which I can pull down over my face. It is very useful when I see one of my father's men."

"If only I'd been able to do that for Bertis." Camdovin's eyes clouded over with sadness. "If only that tough fighter, Lundell, had protected him as he was meant to. Maybe they were taken completely unawares. That's all I can think. You still have a difficult time ahead and it's essential you have trusted protectors with you – two of my men."

"As long as they don't mind travelling by donkey or a donkey-pulled cart!" Kim said smiling, remembering Kelin's warning again.

"Whatever you want you can have!" Camdovin came over and gave him a good pat on the back. "When will you go?" he asked.

"As soon as I can, if you permit."

"How about in three days' time? That will give you time to prepare and to say your goodbyes. The children will miss you and so will Atrell and I."

"And I will miss all of you. But first I have to meet Kelin in the City of Towers. I promised to meet him there in September. He not only saved my life but I owe him money for the maize." Kim also hoped that Kelin would let him continue his journey on horseback. But that was unlikely, because one of the reasons Kelin had said he must ride a donkey was to let people think he was poor and keep the bandits away from him.

He left Camdovin's study with a heavy heart. He had not only got much more to do than he had expected, but there was now a tangible and greater urgency to what he was doing: Sagesse was seriously ill – an anguish he found he could not share with Camdovin. Kim knew that the only way to cure her was to eliminate, by whatever means possible, the power of this curse. There was no doubt in his mind that this evil power was also affecting King Ambab's family, affecting the one person in that family to whom Kim was closest.

Chapter 14
GOODBYES AND A MEETING

The first person he had to see, now, was Tiésa. He wanted to give her back the talisman and to thank her for all her help. Then he would fetch Modo from Sabio and Bava, who had been caring for him all this time.

Tiésa, of course, knew most of what had been going on and now Kim told her everything Camdovin had said and all about the new journey he would have to make to Beran. When he tried to give the talisman back to Tiésa, the old woman wouldn't hear of it.

"Keep it! You still need it. One day you will bring it back to me. When everything has settled down in your life and you have found your heart's desire." Tiésa was laughing now.

"My heart's desire? What do you mean, Tiésa?" exclaimed Kim.

"It's what we all are looking for, and it can be the work of a lifetime. You will find it, Kim, and when you have done that and also found a talisman of your own, then and only then may you return this one to me. And if by any chance I am no longer here, then you can always trust the person who looks after this little shop to know what to do with it. Go and collect Modo now from Bava and her father. They have made good use of him!" With that Kim tied the talisman back into his waistband. Then Tiésa embraced him fondly and waved him on along the road towards Sabio's house.

"Tell him I'll see him later!" She called after him.

That evening, Kim put Modo into one of the stalls with the other donkeys and horses at the Ardair stables. Etsas, the stableman, told him that Camdovin had been asking for him.

When he got to Camdovin's study, the master welcomed Kim.

"How about Erun and Mossim to accompany you?"

Erun and Mossim were the two guards who had been appointed to watch over Kim when he had been imprisoned downstairs in the house. Somewhat to Gralun's annoyance, they had become quite friendly, and Erun had often been found playing chess with Kim in his cell while Mossim kept guard outside.

"That would be very fine!" Kim laughed. "But I only need them as far as the City of Towers. Kelin wanted to meet me there, because he knows a good way past the Vering Mountains, which is virtually bandit free. I shall have a quick overnight stop at Kelin's daughter's farm and will be quite safe after that." Kim told him.

"Well do me a favour, would you? Send one of them back when you meet up with Kelin. But take the other one to Kelin's farm, just so that I don't have to worry! These are expert trained fighters and they can see off any kind of bandit – even if you still insist on travelling by donkey and cart!"

Kim laughed. "Alright," he said. "I think we should dress as poor farmers anyway and put all our provisions into trading sacks."

"That's a good idea …"

"There is one important thing …." Kim tailed off.

"What?"

"It's a great favour I need to ask …" Kim said with some difficulty.

"Ask. I'll do it if I can," said Camdovin with his usual generosity.

"It's to do with one of the kitchen girls. Jisha …" And Kim told Camdovin the story of his own imprisonment in Trasimid jail and his meeting with Lullam; and then he told him Lullam's story. "The trouble is he was imprisoned only because of a corrupt law-officer. But he had no-one important to vouch for his character in court so they didn't believe him. I think Jisha now has serious doubts about whether she was right in not believing her husband. Only, if someone as important as you could help them, I'm sure he will be freed. At least he will be able to have the trust of his family when he does come out of prison."

"I had no idea Jisha was in this situation. She hid it well and it's absolutely my responsibility. I'll see to it," Camdovin said firmly. "The first thing I'll do is have some inquiries made about the officer in question …"

"Thank you, Master," said Kim.

"And don't call me 'Master' any more, will you? You are no longer my servant. We are friends, I think."

* * *

After saying many heartfelt goodbyes – to his two confident and adoring young students, Tamis and Didi; Jisha, to whom he promised that life would soon get a lot better; Tordas and Thovi, the gardeners; and of course, to Atrell, who made him undertake to come back and visit whenever he could – Kim left a few days later with his two companions, Mossim and Erun, for the plains of Memarn where the City of Towers lay. They reckoned it would take a few days to get to the plains and as they got slowly higher, the nights got colder, with daytime still at a comfortable autumnal warmth. In the evenings, after the day's journey, when they had given Modo and the other donkeys grain and hay to eat and had cooked a supper for themselves, they sat in the light of the crumbling fire and played chess.

Erun had carved a set out of the bones he had collected from a butcher he knew. When he and Mossim kept guard, they were allowed a sharp knife in case of attack and at night, or when no-one was about, he had spent time carving the chess pieces. Now, during these cold nights on the plains, the three of them took it in turns to play one another at chess, the third one having the job of cleaning up the pots and pans after supper.

After three days through the hills, they arrived onto the Credairn Plains, the wide, flat area surrounded in the distance by low mountains, with its river running from the Pacelan Mountains to the City of Towers itself, in the middle of the plain.

The towers of its name were six lookout posts placed around the city, tall and with a stark look about them. In the middle of the city was the great square, with its well in the centre where Kim was to meet Kelin.

He had told Kim, "… on the seventh of September, every year for the next three years" … but that was now a good while ago. Kelin had also told him to wait if he was not there on the exact day. But they had arrived a day early, so they were in good time.

They stabled the donkeys, found rooms for themselves and then went to the central square, to a coffee house with a view of the well, five hundred metres away.

"This place is perfect!" Mossim exclaimed. "They have chess tables!" Erun and Mossim could sit and play chess and drink a glass of tea or coffee while waiting for Kim to meet with Kelin.

But Kim was impatient. He hoped he wouldn't have to wait the three days that Kelin had mentioned and he wondered whether he would have the courage to tell him all that had happened and where he was going now. What Kim really needed was to get to Vocimere Palace in Beran's capital as quickly as possible. Would he be able to tell Kelin about Sagesse? He wasn't sure, and today, one day before Kelin was supposed to come, the only person sitting by the well was a young woman.

Kim decided to spend the rest of that day sitting next to the well himself. So he walked over there, leaving the others at the café. He had brought a book with him and when he got near the well, he saw that the young woman was also reading. She didn't look at him at all, but kept on reading, and yet there was something about her – was it her noble profile? – that made him feel strange. They stayed like that for some hours, both sitting quietly on opposite stone benches with the plain trees providing much needed shade and, between them, the well which contained sweet water. Around them people came and went: mothers with their children, old men and young people in groups or alone, all drawn to the promise of a cool drink.

That night, in the room they had found, Kim dreamt that the young woman by the well took off her flowered scarf and he could see that she was unbelievably beautiful. She came up to him as he was hidden in an alcove covered by a thick curtain and she opened the curtain and said, "You must hurry! Your friend is dying. Quick, come quickly! It's simple now because you know the way!" And she led him down dark, winding stairs. When they got to the bottom, she opened the outer door for him and there he was in the countryside.

"Run! Run as fast as you can, otherwise something terrible will happen!" And he ran and ran until he could run no longer.

When Kim awoke, he felt full of fear. Today was September seventh. Please let Kelin come today! he thought.

Now, without warning, he was overcome with a terrible sense of foreboding. What if Kelin wanted to take the talisman? Would he be safe without it? And what if he were to go the rest of the journey by horse? Would he be caught by bandits? He was filled with anxieties.

Would he ever find these papers? Would he be able to get at any legal documents, stored in Vocimere Palace itself, as Camdovin had thought? And the worst, most worrying thought – would he be able to save his beloved Sagesse?

As he approached the well, Kim noticed that the young woman had no book today and she watched him arrive. Then she got up and came towards him.

"Excuse me …" she said politely.

"Hullo …" Kim returned immediately.

"Are you Kim from Derkia, who travelled on the road to Trasimid and visited our friend Tiésa?"

"Yes, I am."

"My name is Habama. I am Kelin's granddaughter."

They shook hands formally.

"Oh … granddaughter …? But why is he not here? Has something happened to him?" Last night's dream flooded back into his mind and he suddenly feared for the safety of the old man. "Is he all right?" Kim asked again.

"He is. He couldn't make the journey this year. He told me to tell you that all is well with him and said I am to lead you through the eastern part of the Vering Mountains by the safe route."

"And you know that route?"

"Yes, I do. My family's been travelling here for around twenty years to sell our produce. Sometimes my father, sometimes all of us, sometimes my grandfather. I have often travelled the route."

"And who did you come with this year?"

"My father. But he had to go on to see someone in the south and he left me here."

"Let me take you to meet the others," said Kim immediately.

"The others?"

"My master in Trasimid insisted I have two companions on my way here. One will return, now that I have met up with you."

"How did you travel?" she asked, moving away from the water well.

"By donkey and cart."

"No horses?"

"No."

"Good. My grandfather said that you must be sure to continue your quest on a donkey. Only if you have succeeded in completing your journey and know everything you need to know, so that all is settled in your life, only then can you go back to riding a horse. That's what he told me to say to you."

Now Kim slowed down his walking. He wanted to ask Habama about the talisman before they reached his chess-playing friends.

"Did he mention a talisman to you?" he asked quietly.

"Yes. He said you must keep the talisman to the end of your journey. And he said your journey does not end when you think it *should* end, but when you *know* it is ended. When everything feels complete, then you can return the talisman to Tiésa. That's what he said."

"That's almost the same as what Tiésa said to me!" Kim laughed. They continued towards Erun and Mossim still playing chess in the café, surrounded by a small group of eager watchers all sitting around them.

* * *

The next day Mossim bought himself a horse, as Camdovin had instructed him. Kim gave him a hug.

"Thank you for all your support," he said to the big man who loved chess. "You made it possible for me to get through those difficult days so full of lies, intrigue and envious malice."

"I could see you weren't quite as bad as they made out." Mossim laughed. "Just a bit of a liar. You don't really come from Grailand, do you?" he went on. "Where are you really from – and why lie about it?"

"I'm really from Strela," said Kim with a twinkle in his eye. "I had a good reason to fib about it and it didn't hurt anyone. But I'll have to tell you that when we next meet; it's a long story." The two gave each other another hug, Mossim said his goodbyes to the others and went on his way, back to his master.

Kim, Habama and Erun now rode on in a north-westerly direction. The route, as Habama explained, was hilly, but it was a path used mostly by shepherds and farmers. Few people knew of its existence and from a bandit's point of view it wasn't worth coming up here except as a getaway. In general, the people on this path had not enough money or riches to be worth robbing.

Their trek over the hills was peaceful and enjoyable; only at night time did Kim return to disturbing dreams –

mainly about Sagesse – leaving him bereft and anxious. One night he called out and woke Habama, who came over to him.

"What is it, Kim? Are you alright?"

"What?" She had awoken him and he was dazed. "Yes. Why? What's the matter?"

"You called out. I think you were asleep."

"It was only a dream … I'm fine." But the dream had shaken him. In the morning he felt better and pleased to continue the journey.

*   *   *

Later that day, going along a narrow pathway, they came across a boy and a man travelling in the same direction, riding a slow, rickety donkey. As they passed the man said, "Have you got any spare food for the donkey? Or some water?" Their donkey looked underfed and decrepit, with the young son clinging to it and his father at the back.

They all stopped in the road and Kim passed some of their precious water in a bucket on to the father and son, who gave it to their donkey. When the water was gone, Habama gave the donkey some grain to eat.

"There's a stream round the next bend and on up a bit," said Habama to the man. "Your donkey will be able to have his fill there."

The man nodded and turned to the boy, putting him up onto the donkey. Then he got up himself, behind the boy. He now hit the donkey several times and it tottered forward uncertainly.

Seeing this, Kim called out, "Hey! Mister!" The man turned around and Kim went on: "Look, we are on our way to the stream too. Why don't you and the boy ride in our cart and let your donkey have a rest?"

"Thank you, sir," said the man. "My donkey's been travelling all day and he's just being lazy now. He can walk behind the cart."

So, for half an hour, Habama, Erun, the man and the boy sat together in the little cart pulled by Camdovin's two donkeys and followed by the farmer's thin, sad donkey, with Kim ahead on Modo. Rounding a corner, the path went sharply upwards for a little and then dipped down, towards a bubbling stream. There was a spurt as the donkeys, hearing running water, made a dash forward.

In a moment they were, all of them – men, girl, boys and animals – drinking thirstily at the stream. Only the sad little donkey moved half-heartedly towards the water, until his master gave him a lashing with a stick. Kim saw this from the corner of his eye as he was drinking and, as Kim got up, he could see the donkey move towards the stream and drink with the others. But it was followed by the man and even though the donkey was now drinking, the man started beating it again. The donkey seemed to ignore the lashings onto its bony backside.

"Hey! What are you doing?" Kim shouted, as he watched all this, now in a fury and running to where the man was.

The others looked up in surprise as Kim reached the man and tried to grab hold of his stick.

"You can't do that!" Kim shouted at the man, succeeding in snatching the stick from him. "The donkey didn't harm you!"

"He needs to do what I tell him!" said the man angrily, trying to pull the stick away from Kim. "He never does what he's told!"

"That's because you beat him, so he doesn't see any point. Look at the marks on him!" Kim, still holding the stick, was inspecting the donkey now.

"It's none of your business! He's my donkey!" The man shouted, trying to get his stick back again. Man and boy now started a tussle for the stick and soon Kim, in an explosion of rage, had the man pinned down on the ground.

"How would you like to be half-starved and then beaten for no reason?" Kim yelled at the man. "You're not fit to own an animal if that's how you treat a helpless creature!" Kim was so enraged he could barely keep himself from throttling the man. Finally, Erun rushed up and pulled Kim off him while Habama comforted the boy, who was now very upset.

"Come on," Erun was saying to Kim, "calm down … He didn't hurt the donkey that much …"

"He was pushing it and beating it for no reason! And anyway, look at the poor creature. It's half-starved. That donkey's probably so hardened to beatings," he turned back to the man, "he doesn't even care any longer! He probably wants you to kill him, rather than be tortured like this!" Kim was still beside himself shouting at the man and trying to get out of Erun's firm hold. "I suppose you bully and beat your children too, tell them that they're useless and worthless good-for-nothings who waste your energy! I suppose you tell them that too!"

"Calm down, Kim," said Erun, still restraining him.

The little boy was now watching intently as his father picked himself up and walked towards his donkey, pulling the animal away from the stream where he'd been drinking. The boy moved towards his father, but out of reach of him, going the opposite side of the skinny donkey as the man pulled it up the path.

The man then put his son onto the donkey and pulled himself up behind him and they all moved off, down the path, with the donkey looking extremely fragile, carrying its human load.

"That animal's going to collapse at any moment," moaned Kim, watching them go. Erun had let Kim go by now and Kim was fuming again. "There should be a law against such maltreatment!"

"Yes, that's true. But it doesn't warrant such a barrage of anger," said Erun. "What got into you? I've never seen you like that before."

"Sorry," said Kim sheepishly. "I can get very upset when there's an injustice. I just somehow go berserk. I don't know why."

"Perhaps we should buy the donkey from the man," suggested Habama, who was also distressed at the sight of the stricken animal. "Then we might be able to nurse it back to health ... You have enough money, don't you?" she said, turning to Kim. "Ninety crowns should be more than enough."

"Go on," Kim said to her, giving her a one hundred piece, "try and persuade him!"

Habama ran off immediately to catch up with the departing trio.

"Hey mister!" she called. "Hey mister, and your son! We've got an offer to make to you!" She caught up with them and Kim could see her talking animatedly, while the man and boy listened. After a moment, without any fuss, they both got off the donkey and all three stood there looking at it. The next moment Habama was handing over the money to the man and then man and boy walked off, having given the donkey's rope to Habama. Now she walked slowly back towards Kim and Erun, leading the donkey back to the stream to let him drink again; she picked some choice grass for him to eat and quietly stroked his neck. At first, he shook her away, fearing this new treatment. But Habama persisted and, as he ate, she continued to stroke him gently.

Then they roped the donkey – which Habama had found out was called Xoni – to the back of the cart and continued on their way. By the time they reached the farm belonging to Murima, Kelin's daughter, where Kelin was staying, Xoni had already become slightly plumper and a lot less nervous.

* * *

They were greeted at the door by Kelin. "How wonderful to see you!" he exclaimed with delight, giving Kim a hug. "I do believe you have grown an inch or two!" he laughed. And after introductions had been made, they were led into the cottage, where the hungry travellers were happy to see what looked like a big feast being set onto the table. This went on well into the night. Kim was able to give Kelin the money for the maize he had sold, which they had agreed on, as well as the newly strengthened Xoni as a gift and the other two donkeys to replace Modo, who Kim had grown so fond of.

Kim told them about his adventures in Trasimid and joked a lot about his imprisonment in Camdovin's house. Later he explained privately to Kelin all about his mission and why it had been so important for him to find Camdovin and even how he had seen several of his father's men looking for him.

"Well, your father's men certainly won't find you on the road I'm going to show you, near the Vering Mountains, because it is known only to locals. They're more likely to be looking for you in Beran than in the countryside. So please take great care and keep wearing my old hat!" Kelin advised.

The next day, after Erun had found a horse and amid hugs and gratitude, he, in his turn, went on his way back to Ardair.

Kim stayed another day with his old friend and saviour; he knew he could wait no longer to find out more about Sagesse and search for Camdovin's papers. So the next day, riding on Modo, he made his way north towards Beran, to find the notes that Camdovin had written all those years ago and which he had hidden in the Vocimere Palace oak tree.

* * *

The route Kelin had told him about led around the Vering Mountains, through the foothills, on the way to Sendrala, at the Gean Sea. The mountains themselves were notoriously high and difficult. Going over them would take him too long and tire Modo out unnecessarily.

Instead, he went southeast, along the northwest of Memarn itself, leading to the port of Sendrala on the Gean Sea, with its high, jutting ramparts, its inlets, islands and bridges.

Still as unobtrusive as possible for fear of his father's men, Kim and Modo took a ferryboat across the Gean Sea, straight to the harbour city of Eider, in Beran, and from there north to Sarsi. Inside that great fortified city, with its hills around, stood Vocimere Palace.

Chapter 15
HIDDEN TREASURE

On arriving in Sarsi, Kim immediately took Modo to stay in a nearby stable and then rented a room for himself. He found the marketplace, which he had never visited before, and a little corner shop which sold things like large hats, long canes and walking sticks and – what he was looking for – a large, dark, hooded cloak.

That night, wondering if he had managed to lose his father's men now that he was away from Trasimid, Kim left his room and made his way in the dark, up the hill towards the palace. He had only ever been inside the grounds so had never seen it properly from the outside. It took a bit of working out to know where he was in relation to the gardens. There was a high wall all around and eight gates within that wall, except for the main entrance to the palace which had its own special, large gate and a wide drive up to the main entrance of the palace. At each gate a guard stood solemnly by with his sword. He didn't want to inspect them as he was wary of being noticed, so after a little look he went back to his room.

How am I going to get into the grounds? Kim thought to himself. One way could be to scale the wall in between the regular gates, if I find somewhere the guards can't see me.

His mother had made it clear that this quest was secret, meaning that King Ambab and his family, as well as everyone else except for Camdovin, must not know about it until it was completed. But there was also another urgency which she hadn't known about: Sagesse's illness. So, however tempting it was to talk to them, if any of the Beran royal family found out even a little bit about what he was doing, it could jeopardise the whole of his mission, especially as Camdovin had thought King Ambab *might* possibly have been knowingly involved in all this.

Time was of the essence, Kim knew, but he would absolutely have to see the layout of the palace wall again.

The next night, Kim went again to the palace wall to inspect it from a slight distance. He took care guards didn't see what he was doing and pretended to be delivering a package nearby. He discovered one part of the wall where guards on either side could not see him. It seemed the one blind-spot. This was where he would try to scale the wall. On this side of the palace there were no buildings, but fields and stables further away. There was often activity at the stables, even at night, only it was far away enough not to interfere with the night-time peace and silence of the road around the palace. Unless there was a very bright moon, Kim would be almost invisible both from the stables and from the guards.

Luckily on the next night there were only a few thin clouds, with the moonlight showing brightly through them. Having donned the cloak, which covered him entirely, he made his way over to that side of the palace wall with his rope and hook.

Kim had memorised the layout of the gardens; after all, he had played hide and seek there often enough. He knew the hollow oak was at a point halfway between the outer wall and the palace and he remembered Camdovin's words: "Inside, there is just enough room for a man and there's a kind of bench. At about two metres high, well above the entrance to the hollow, there's another smaller ledge." That's what Kim must find. But would the oak tree still be there after all this time?

From the road, carefully making sure that he was out of sight of any guards, Kim threw the hook and rope up onto the top of the wall. It made a bit of a crack, but he waited flat against the wall and no-one came running. Then he climbed up it as quickly as he could.

At the top of the wall, he threw his hooked rope down and jumped soundlessly onto the soft, mossy grass. Leaving the rope where he could find it again, Kim ran left along the sheltering darkness of the inside edge of the wall until he came to one of the paths leading straight to the palace. He turned right now, along the path. Here, he needed to look out for the tree.

I'm sure it's a little way to the right of this path, but the question is how far to the right, and will I see it in this darkness? he asked himself. Every time he came to a tree he felt around its trunk for a hollow; but they were all solid.

After over half an hour of doing this, and having strayed now a long way from the original path, Kim realised he was completely lost.

The thing is, would it be wiser to wait until it's light to find the tree, or go back and come again tomorrow? But then tomorrow night I will have the same difficulty finding the tree as I'm having now! he thought.

Making sure there was no gateway nearby, Kim stumbled back to the wall and sat down to wait for first light. He guessed it was now well past one o'clock and he dozed a little.

After what seemed like only twenty minutes, he began to see the dark silhouette of Vocimere Palace looming up behind the trees as the sky became lighter. When he could see better, he got up and moved silently towards the palace to get his bearings. That way he would definitely find the tree.

Now he realised that he had entered the palace grounds further to the west than he had imagined, so back at the wall he crept along to the right, found the path he needed and moved into it near to where he thought the tree was. He was now moving easily in the pre-dawn light towards the oak tree. It was still dark enough for him to be invisible from the palace, he thought. But he was surprised how completely different the garden looked from this side and how difficult it was to see where the tree actually was. Perhaps it had been cut down in the meantime, he worried. Maybe after all these years it was simply that everything had grown.

Suddenly he came upon the oak, as if by chance. It was still there, as inviting as it used to be, the ground around it covered now in more moss. He breathed in the scent of flowers that always pervaded it and hauled himself inside. He smelled the early morning damp on the inside of this ancient oak and touched around the hollowed-out trunk. Then he moved his hands up, facing towards the outside. Camdovin had said the ledge was well above his head. As Kim moved both hands upwards, he felt something hard and slimy. When he pulled it, it came away. It was a metal box, not large, but covered in moss. Camdovin had mentioned no metal box. He had just said a roll of papers in leather.

Kim scraped off the moss with his fingers and wiped it with his cloak. He climbed out of the tree and now, hidden by the trees and in near daylight, he opened it. Inside was the leather, wrapping up a roll. Kim unravelled it and there were the notes, as Camdovin had said, written in a careful, youthful hand. Five pages of two sides, Kim counted. He rolled them back into the leather, put the roll in the box, put the box into a large pocket of his cloak, then ran silently back to the outer wall.

He would wait here all day now and find the place he had dropped his rope later, when it was dark. Here he was well hidden from anyone looking out of a window. This area of the grounds was more heavily wooded than towards the palace; near the wall it was dark and shaded, even in the sunlight. It was only rarely that they, as children, had ever come this far, playing their games; also, while playing "hide and seek" they had kept away from the dank, mossy, dark green area by the wall.

Kim lay down, wrapped himself into his cloak and prepared to sleep.

* * *

He awoke suddenly. The sun was shining overhead, though of course he was hidden. The sound of children's voices was clear in his ears. Had he dreamt them? Was it a memory? Then the sound came again, loud and clear. "Look!" It was a girl's voice.

"What?" came a boyish voice.

"Look what I can see!"

"Don't go near there. They told us not to go far into the trees!" came the boy's voice again.

"But look, Ravi!" came the girl's voice again. "There's someone's boot!"

"Don't be silly!" the boy insisted.

But Kim's boot was completely visible as, while he was sleeping, he had stretched his leg out of the vegetation by the wall.

Instinctively, he pulled it back, out of sight.

"Where is it?" the boy asked.

"Over there," she said. Then: "Oh! It's gone …"

"You're just making it up."

"No! It was there" the girl insisted. "I really did see it."

"Well, it can't have moved on its own. Do you think there's a person there?"

"I only saw a boot."

"I'm going to have a look. You stay there," said the boy gallantly. But the little girl followed closely behind him, as the boy went slowly and carefully towards where the girl had pointed.

Kim held his breath. Would they find him? The

children were getting closer and he had nowhere to run except along the wall. He quickly tried to work out where he had left the rope; he was almost sure it was now to the right of him, but he was not *absolutely* sure. Should he make a run for it, or should he beg the children not to tell? After all, he was doing no harm to anyone. But he knew to his cost that fact was no guarantee of his safety! Suddenly he realised that the children were not going to help him. Why should they? They didn't know who he was. If he had to go to the palace at any time later, they – whoever these children were – might recognise him. Still, the little boy was plodding determinedly towards where he was hiding. He couldn't risk it.

The next moment, with a cry of fright from the two children, Kim jumped up with a swoosh, and was running along the wall, his great black cloak trailing up behind him like a giant bat's wings. If the guards saw him, he would simply run for it. As to reading Camdovin's secret notes, that must wait until he reached his room.

He found the rope and swung it over the top of the wall, scaling it with a speed he'd never imagined he had, with Camdovin's notes stashed inside the pocket of his cloak. On the other side of the wall, he simply left his rope and ran. He could hear the guards talk and then some shouting, but he was away and out of sight now and quickly shed his cloak, carrying it rolled up as a bundle, under his arm.

In his room he found some bread and cheese and ate it ravenously, calming his nerves. He was both afraid and excited about what he would read. Would this be, at last, the answer to all his problems? Would he finally know the secret of the curse?

Kim opened the box gently, took out the leather roll and unwound it. He pulled out the batch of papers and tried to flatten them, but they remained curled, resisting his intrusion after so long a time. What would he find? He bent them determinedly the other way around and started to read.

By me, Balquin, kitchen boy. What I heard at the top of the stairs in Koremine Castle, Strela, in year ----:

In the room there were Prince Callouste, Prince Demble, King Strearn and Queen Porla. I was sent up on an errand and found myself hiding behind a curtain next to the large library, where the four of them were quarrelling.

IT SEEMED TO ME THAT QUEEN PORLA WAS ALMOST HYSTERICAL DURING THIS ROW.

STREARN:	*I knew about it!*
PORLA:	*You knew? And you let these two … I have given birth to two criminals – murderers!*
DEMBLE:	*We've never killed anyone!*
PORLA:	*You failed to stop the people being killed! You poisoned them!*
STREARN:	*Calm down, Porla!*
PORLA:	*No! My sons are murderers!*
DEMBLE:	*Mother! For God's sake! I don't think Ambab even noticed …*

CALLOUSTE:	*Ambab was in on it anyway …*
STREARN:	*I thought you said he didn't know about it!*
DEMBLE:	*He didn't. His chief accountant was easy to bribe. Ambab never looked at the figures.*
PORLA:	*I don't believe what I am hearing! You two are like petty criminals, gloating over a bad deed … And why? Why? Because you don't care who you steal from! If you, at the top of the scale, can do something like that, no wonder there's so much banditry and theft in the southern borders!*
STREARN:	*This deal with Kardra and Co. was the only place they could get the money from! What were they supposed to do?*
PORLA:	*And what was the result of their greed?*

HERE I THINK SHE BURST INTO TEARS.

STREARN:	*They had to get the money from somewhere!*
PORLA:	*What do other people do in that position if they run out of money? They don't poison people or allow them to die!*
STREARN:	*The only thing to do is sell some of their treasures …*
PORLA:	*If you're lucky enough to have treasures …*

STREARN: But Demble and Callouste couldn't do that!

PORLA: Why couldn't they?

SHE WAS IN A TOTAL FURY.

STREARN: Those treasures don't belong to them, they belong to me – to the whole family, not just to them!

PORLA: You prevented them selling our treasures! It was you who let them steal from people who were already poor and starving. You who should set an example as the king.

STREARN: It was never our intention to poison people.

PORLA: What happens if you take safeguards away from the drinking water and the water becomes contaminated? People die when their water is contaminated. You knew that!

STREARN: They found a way out of their difficulties which didn't upset anyone important …

PORLA: Anyone important!

AND HERE SHE SET UP HER SCREAMING AGAIN

PORLA: Are the people of our country not important? Are they simply a vehicle for you and your sons' excesses! It led directly to the lack of clean water in the south and lack of medicines when the children were ill! They were *dying because we couldn't afford the remedies! Children were dying! There was poisoned water and people couldn't water their crops! And all you worry about is that it didn't affect important people!*

DEMBLE: *Mother! Please calm down, mother!*

PORLA: *What is your job? Your work, Strearn? Is it to keep yourself in riches and treasures, or is it to look after the people of your country?*

CALLOUSTE: *Mother, please don't shriek! Please!*

PORLA: *Answer me that question! Is it to look after yourselves?*

STREARN: *Don't make so much noise, Porla! The whole castle will hear what you're saying!*

PORLA: *When we are so wealthy compared to most people in the land, all you can think about is getting richer! And at their cost!*

STREARN: *If we are in trouble, how can we be of any use in the land?*

PORLA: *Because of your taking money from funds that were meant to keep people healthy – because of all that, the cook's whole family died. People we know! The stable boy, his mother died. The coachman! Yes! Purmis, his sister and three of her children died. Do you even care? The kitchen boy, Balquin's parents perished. And all because of you, Strearn, with your two sons – taking funds that were allotted to medicines for water, and for food in case of emergency! You killed them! What kind of king are you?*

I had heard enough. I was suddenly in pain listening to this as I had been in terrible pain a few years before, when both my parents had died from poisoned water and an infection, impossible to cure because we did not have the medicines. Many in my village had died. My closest friend, Bawan, and the girl I wanted to marry, Lecia, had all died. I was left utterly bereft.

I jumped from the cubby hole and ran down as quickly as I could. When I got to the kitchen, I was shaking all over. I told them that they were quarrelling about money and that it seemed that Prince Demble and Prince Callouste had done something bad, though I wasn't sure what it was. I could barely talk and, in the end, they took me to my bed hoping I'd be better the next day. It took me months to get rid of the shakes completely. Some days later Queen Porla was found dead. It was said she died of shock and grief, but no-one knew why. Though I know that people can get ill and die when they have a shock, I believe it was her husband and two sons who killed her, though maybe not deliberately. But I was not sure whether her death had a more sinister cause.

I became fearful that my own life would be in danger if anyone knew that I had heard the quarrel and what was said. So, I decided to run away, to escape and find a new life in *another country.*

On my way, I have written down what I heard as nearly as possible, and will hide it away for anyone who might have need of it.

There must be documents held by King Ambab, or his heirs, from Kardra and Company about transactions; these would show up the truth of the terrible fraud which caused the contamination, and thus verify the truth of these words.

And the papers were signed at the end:

Balquin of the village of Jusas, Strela, with a date.

* * *

Kim sat in a daze. His own father had been the deliberate cause of the death of, amongst many, many others, Camdovin's parents. And all for the sake of having a lavish lifestyle.

He wanted to weep, to show some feeling of solidarity with the horrifically deprived of his own country. But tears would not come. He felt drained and emotionless. His heart felt icy and if he had been near his father at this moment, he would have gladly killed him.

Only he was not near his father. In this room, he was not near anyone; even Modo was away in a stable.

He slept until five o'clock the next day and then ran out in time to buy some food at the market. At a corner stall, the sight of bright flowers made him think again of dear Modo, whom he knew would love to have a munch of these.

Two stallholders were talking nearby. "They say she's

no better than a month ago," said the first stallholder.

"The palace is asking for people to bring special herbs because she's taken a turn for the worse," answered the second. "One of the physicians thinks she won't last another month, if she goes on deteriorating at this rate."

"I wouldn't know which herbs to take her," said the first, looking at his flowers and bunches of dried herbs.

"Maybe Fava will know. I'll find out if she can help our lovely princess."

Kim stared. Sagesse had taken a turn for the worse and may not last, and he had barely got hold of anything to get rid of the curse – this curse that his father, uncle and grandfather had put onto their own family and anyone connected to it, and also onto the whole land of Strela and its people. Sagesse preyed on his mind unrelentingly. How could he prevent her from succumbing further to illness still with so much to do? How would he do it in time? One month! If only Tiésa were here to help her. But no, it was up to Kim to complete his task immediately, in secrecy and before any of his father's men caught up with him. There was no other way but to do something similar with King Ambab as he had done with Camdovin: get work at the palace.

Chapter 16
IN VOCIMERE PALACE

Kim needed the proof of what his father, uncle and grandfather had done to cause this curse; once he had that, broadcasting it about, if necessary, would be the solution. He believed Tiésa when she said that one of the most powerful ways to get rid of a bad deed was to tell it to all and sundry; that took the power away from any secret curse. If it was an evil deed which was also against the law, the law should be meted out to the criminal.

Kim fervently hoped the proof could be found in the accounting offices of the palace, where King Ambab had almost certainly stored records of the Kardra & Co. transactions. At the same time, however much he would have liked to confide in Sagesse or King Ambab himself, he knew he couldn't do so. Until he had all the facts in his hands, secrecy was a necessity for breaking the spell. He would have to continue on his own until he got hold of the information somehow. But how?

He and Camdovin had discussed methods of getting into the palace. The best way would be with a personal recommendation and Camdovin had given him separate letters saying that he was competent in a few different fields: secretarial, clerical, basic accounting, also mentioning the tutoring of his children. The first three were areas of work that seemed more likely to give Kim access to the documents he needed. In other letters Camdovin praised his ability with plants, as a sportsman, and lastly as a kitchen worker. But because the documents Kim needed were related to business and accounting, it would clearly be most useful for him to get work in that department.

Kim now wrote a letter to the palace under the name "Distrell", a name he and Camdovin had decided on, asking for work in the accounts department.

Dear sir, he wrote, *I am writing to you because I wondered if you have need of a clerk in your accounting department. I have worked principally with the Master of Building and Trading, Camdovin, in Memarn, and he has given me a letter of recommendation …*

"Now is the time for a change," Kim thought. He went out and bought a good wig which he fixed well below his hairline to change the shape of his face; then he cut the beard which he had grown, leaving only a moustache, which he trained down over his lips to hide the true line of his mouth. His build was anyway more athletic than it had been – he had lost the puppy-fat of a year ago – and he bought some dark shadowing to put around his eyes, making them look deeper set and his face bonier. But he liked the result and to complete the picture he bought a new outfit, immediately fixing the ever-present talisman into the waistband. Looking in the mirror, Kim was pleased.

"It doesn't look like me at all!" No-one would recognise him.

After two days Kim got a reply from the palace asking him to come to see them the following week.

He decided now to change another aspect of himself: his gait. He would adopt a different way of walking and moving, so that if the other two things failed, his movements and walk would look so totally unlike the Prince Kim they had seen, that they would be certain this was a person who simply looked a bit like him. He fitted slivers of wood into the instep of each shoe so that he walked on the outside of his feet, making him walk in a bow-legged fashion, with his legs looking slightly curved.

Although his facial expression was changed now because of the moustache and he looked much older than his young years, he resolved to imagine himself as a different character, to act like a small-minded man, finicky, humourless, slightly vain and interested in nothing other than his work. He tightened his voice and practised reading the letter aloud to himself. He put himself into his new clothes and spent time walking around his room, getting used to the uncomfortable shoes and the gait of someone older.

He moved to a new room, taking it on as "Distrell", and he now became this man as much as possible. He even made one or two acquaintances as *Distrell*.

If Kim, as Distrell, managed to pass the interview, he would be able to offer himself as a clerk of the best quality. Camdovin had often given him clerk's duties and Kim knew the ropes well enough. This was the job that would get him near to the business workings of King Ambab. His only fear was that he might also find himself confronted with the king himself.

Eventually, having made up and learned by heart a new history and clutching Camdovin's letter, which related to a man called Distrell, he presented himself at Vocimere Palace. At the gate he showed the letter he had received from them and, going through the driveway, he recalled the last time he had been here, and felt again a terrible longing to see Sagesse.

The serious-faced, thin man who received him in the hallway shook his hand solemnly, introduced himself as Glendor and took him to a nearby chamber as Kim handed him Camdovin's letter.

"Please sit down," said Glendor, and he started to read the letter. Kim looked about him. It was a simply furnished room with a window onto the gardens. He withstood the temptation to look out to see where he had hidden just a few days ago. The character he was now, Distrell, was taciturn and passive; he would not offer information he had not been asked for and he would not, at present, show much interest in anything.

"Well," said Glendor when he had finished reading, "so, Camdovin, eh? He's got a good reputation abroad. He seems to have liked you, but I should tell you that we are looking for the right person, rather than just anyone to fill the post quickly." He looked briefly at the letter again and went on, "I would like you to meet our chief accountant, Mr Olban. Would you be able to come tomorrow?"

"Certainly," responded Kim.

So Kim, as Distrell, found himself a day later in another interview at the palace. He portrayed carefully his "retiring, but able" clerk's personality and found after this second interview that he was asked to join the palace staff.

Kim now kept his head down, working hard, quickly learning the ropes and giving out an aura of insignificant trustworthiness. People ignored him if possible; he was liked for his hard work and unobtrusiveness, and relied upon because he was mediocre.

But he was impatient and worried constantly about Sagesse. One day, in the canteen, two maids were gossiping loudly at the end of the table where Kim had sat down.

"They say you can't rely on what she is going to be like: one moment sweet as pie, the next a vicious roaring lion," said the maid sitting nearest Kim.

"She's got so thin now you would never recognise her. Pale as a ghost. Well, you know she'll only eat a kind of gruel," said the other, opposite her.

"I heard she would only eat sweetmeats!"

"And she writes poetry all the time, while crying and suffering from agora-something … doesn't dare go outside her room."

"Agoraphobia?"

"Yes. She won't see anyone, you know … Oh! I must fetch those pies …! Cook will kill me!" And the second maid rushed off, leaving the first maid to finish her lunch in silence, with Kim sitting, shocked and perplexed, at the other end of the table. Were these stories just gossip? The worst of it was that Kim's thoughts now centred around Sagesse and not on the urgent task which would free her: the finding of those important documents.

A few evenings later, Kim was feeling particularly dejected as he walked home along a quiet street. He looked up at the moon and thought: this is the same moon that Sagesse can see from her window – we can both look at it. Further down the street, a lone man walked towards him. As the man got nearer, Kim realised it was Pelo, one of his father's men. But there was nowhere here to hide or run! And worse, as they passed, Kim caught his eye and they exchanged looks; there was absolutely no chance that Pelo hadn't seen him.

Kim averted his eyes as quickly as he could, hoping and praying that Pelo wouldn't have recognised him through his disguise. Thank God! Pelo passed him by without any recognition and Kim continued on at the same pace.

The next moment there was a shout. "Excuse me!"

Kim turned slowly in fear. Was he going to stop him now? Would he have to run for it? With bits of wood in his shoes? He would never outrun Pelo!

"Are you addressing me, sir?" Kim asked in Distrell's squeaky voice.

"Yes. I wondered if you know where Serda Street is?" Pelo replied.

"I think it may be the second or third on the left, that way, but I'm not from this district."

"Thank you," the army man said and Kim turned

and walked slowly on his way, breathing as slowly as he could but tempted to run even with the pieces of wood in his shoes. Why did he have such an urge to run? Did Pelo suspect? Had he noticed something? Instead, Kim, now at some distance from Pelo, turned to see how far away Pelo was – whether he had moved away as swiftly as it seemed he would. To Kim's horror, Pelo was standing stock still, almost in the same place Kim had left him. Pelo was staring at him in disbelief.

He knows, Kim thought. He knows who you are! Keep the same rhythm in your walking, but larger, longer paces, he told himself in a panic. You might be able to make that turning before he runs after you. Then take the wood out of your shoes and run for it. Hide if you see somewhere to hide – a hedge, a tree – anything.

All these thoughts rushed through Kim's head and he quickened his pace and reached the corner of the next road and rounded it. He quickly slipped the pieces of wood from his shoes and ran, with all the speed he could muster, then crouched right down behind a tree in a garden and watched.

A moment later Pelo appeared at the corner, looking around him, seeing nothing, and deciding it must have been a mistake. He would talk to the general tomorrow morning about what he had seen. After all, it couldn't be that the young Prince Kim would look so different and although it was a while since anyone had seen him, he couldn't have changed that much – could he? And yet ... The thoughts lingered on in Pelo's mind as he made his way back to his base.

*   *   *

A few days later, as Kim was sitting at his desk writing out some kitchen accounts, Glendor came in and told him that Olban needed him to sort something out in the accounts' library. Kim's heart took a leap.

"When you've finished, go to Olban's office. He'll tell you what needs to be done."

At Olban's office, he was sent to the second floor, third door along, on the right.

"What am I to do there?" asked Kim, as blankly as he could.

"I want you to find the accounts for two years ago, looking for the specific amount of five hundred and thirty-six cudres."

"Paid to ...?"

"Paid to a contract in Strela. Dulam and Co. It's on the left as you go in, but it could take you sometime." Kim's heart was thumping, but he was watching the chief accountant carefully as he opened the drawer in front of him and took out a key.

Kim knew that to search for the twenty-four-year-old papers of Kardra & Co. he needed could take him all night. But now he would take as long as possible on Olban's Dulam & Co. file to find out the workings of this accounts library and discover exactly where he should look for the old Kardra documents that Camdovin had cited.

Once in the accounts' library, he looked around to see how secluded a place it was. If he were to hide here, would he be able to put much light in here without being seen from outside? No. There was a large window with inside shutters. But he could use one or two candles.

He needed two sets of documents: the Kardra payments and the discrepancies with the taxes. Camdovin had mentioned two actual years when this fraud could have occurred, he hadn't been sure.

After three quarters of an hour Kim came to a file headed *"Documents, Land Covenants, Taxations and Reforms, Number 1"* and the year was given. He found nine files there, so he guessed that it would not take more than one night to go through. Thank God! Now he concentrated on Mr Olban's work and found, with comparative ease, the Dulam & Co. folder.

The very next day, after work, Kim went to the nearest set of toilets and hid there, waiting until everyone had gone home. When all was quiet, he crept out of the cabin and went to Olban's office, praying that no-one would be there. It was still quiet as he got to Olban's desk and opened the drawer with the key in it.

Then he heard voices.

Was it Olban, back again for something? He waited, immobile. What would he say? But no, it was women's voices and they were walking towards the offices with mops and brooms in their hands.

As the door opened into Olban's office, Kim was on his way towards it, clutching in one hand, tightly, the key to the accounts' library and in the other a bunch of papers which he waved at the two women.

"Stupidly, I forgot these!" And he rushed past them in a terrible hurry.

Down on the second floor Kim entered the third door along with his newly acquired key, locked it behind him, took the keys out of the door and went to sit behind a shelf to eat the food he had brought. Then he dozed off, until this wing of the palace was completely silent. The royal family lived in another part of the palace and oh, he so wished he could just go and see Sagesse. But he knew he couldn't. Luckily, this floor, where he was now, seemed to consist mainly of storerooms.

Kim then stuck some paper along the bottom of the door so that light would not show through, closed the shutters as silently as he could and lit his candles. Then he set to work.

By two-thirty in the morning, he had found two different documents regarding medicines and water purity in Strela. All he needed now was to find a third document, to clinch it. In that year, at the time of flooding and water contamination, cures for the ordinary people in southern Strela had *not* been provided, causing illness and death everywhere. One paper about Strela that he found made it clear that funds had been cancelled *after* the catastrophic contamination had happened, when it was already known that there was a desperate need in Strela. On the other hand, in Beran where there was similar flooding and water contamination, King Ambab *had* provided the necessary funds for medicines.

Then, just after three in the morning, Kim came across the third document. This one was more incriminating. It referred specifically to the Princes Demble and Callouste, saying that revenues and income, jointly agreed with

King Ambab, had to be repaid by the 17 November of that year. Kim looked through but there was nothing to show that this large sum had been given back. The refunding of that amount would have been to the benefit of both countries and their peoples. King Ambab must simply have assumed it had been paid, thought Kim, relieved that it looked as if King Ambab, at least, was innocent of the crime.

After he had kept out the relevant papers and as Kim was putting the files back into the shelves, he heard the sound of footsteps outside in the corridor. He froze. Then quickly he blew out the candles. Who could it possibly be at this time? And why on this floor? He hadn't made any noise.

Silently, he lifted the documents and the candle-lamps off the table and moved to his hiding place. The footsteps reached outside the door, then stopped. The person would need a key to get in. Kim stopped breathing. Would the key turn in the lock? He heard a bunch of keys rattling. Yes, there it was, slowly turning. Who on earth? Why on earth?

Kim was motionless, still holding his breath. A man's voice came softly, whispering to himself: "Funny smell in here. I must get the cleaners to have a good go. Left the shutters closed, maybe that's why it smells ..."

The man, who Kim could just espy through the shelves of files, moved to the window and opened the shutters. He looked around cursorily and then left the room without noticing the paper taped over the bottom of the door.

As Kim heard the lock turn in the door again, he let out a slow sigh. Phew! Thank God the man had not looked more carefully around this little accounts' library, or he would have found a shaking "Distrell" sitting on the floor holding some warm candles and a bunch of papers. Kim would no doubt have been hauled before King Ambab and forced to confess everything. But he wasn't quite ready. He had a few more things to do here, secretly, in Vocimere Palace.

Kim waited in the silent darkness. He had what he needed. All he had to do now was to get out, put the key back in Olban's drawer and sit in the toilet for a few hours until it started up again in the morning. Then he'd walk into the office as if he'd just come from home.

After half an hour Kim was sure he could leave. He took his bag with the papers, pulled the strip from the bottom of the door and slowly and as quietly as possible, unlocked the door. All was silent. He stood there for a minute waiting to hear if the man was anywhere near, but there was no sound whatsoever.

With his shoes in his hand, his documents in his bag and Olban's key in his pocket, Kim ran silently up the stairs to the third floor. There was not a soul as he moved quickly into Olban's office, put back the key and ran out again.

Chapter 17
KING AMBAB GETS A SHOCK

When Kim had first arrived at the palace as an accountant's clerk, he'd assumed he would leave the palace as soon as he had found the documents. But now that he was here and realised how ill Sagesse was, he knew it was crucial she recover very soon, otherwise she may not survive. The trouble was that because of what his mother had said, he must effect a cure in secret. This was an urgent matter and on top of it, he sensed his father's men closing in. Pelo would search for the man he had seen; Kim was sure of it. The men would all be brought to Sarsi and being a small city, it would be much easier to find Kim than in Trasimid – possibly before he'd had the chance to speak to the king. And yet he knew Sagesse's health depended on the secrecy that he had promised his mother. Sagesse must be well before Kim spoke to her father and, of course, before his father's men succeeded in finding him.

In the interview, Glendor had asked Kim what his interests were. He had said gardening. After a few weeks, when he had proved himself as a trustworthy worker, he had asked Glendor if it was permitted for employees to go into the gardens.

"Certain parts are permitted," Glendor had answered. "The north and east parts, because those areas are only rarely used by guests and the family."

"Only I have an interest in gardening and nature, and I have seen some beautiful trees there, in particular an acacia. I would love to have a look at it if I may." But Glendor had made some noncommittal reply and they had left it.

Later Glendor sent Kim down on an unusual errand into the kitchen: a query about a number of eggs.

"You can have a look at that tree, if you hurry!" Glendor had joked. "It's near the kitchens!" He was in a good mood today and Kim took advantage of it. After sorting out the correct quantity of eggs with the chief cook, Kim took his way round to the gardens.

He knew the way, but he'd do things the way Glendor suggested. He walked to the part of the garden where the old hollow oak was, but pretended to look at the exceptionally beautiful acacia nearby. Then, walking back near the oak, he dropped something. As he picked it up, he also pocketed two handfuls of nuts which he found hidden under the moss around the oak tree. Then he strolled back, surprised and delighted by various trees on his way back.

From then on, he bored everyone in the office with talk about the garden, so that soon he was given a special, unspoken licence to visit the gardens whenever possible – given partly in the hope of keeping him quiet.

Meanwhile, a small, anonymous package arrived at the palace for Sagesse. Rania, her maid was with her when it came.

"It's marked, *'For Princess Sagesse: a cure'*. Fancy that! Maybe it's from one of those herbal people your father's been trying to get hold of."

"Let me see," said Sagesse, opening the little box. "Oh look!"

Rania laughed when she saw what was inside. But Sagesse immediately found something to break the shells with and ate them all up.

"It can't do me any harm," she said, as her maid watched her in surprise, noticing that Sagesse seemed to become less frightened.

Ten days after that, Sagesse's maid came to her door again, this time holding a vase with some little flowers in it. She kept knocking until at last, the voice of Sagesse came from inside, "Come in. It's not locked!"

"Oh, Your Highness, I'm so sorry, I thought it was locked." Rania was quite flustered.

"No, Rania. I've stopped locking the doors."

"I think those hazelnuts really did you good then, didn't they?"

"They did."

Then Rania handed Sagesse the vase of flowers she had brought.

"Here are some flowers picked by I-don't-know-who, and sent up in a hurry. There is a message with them." And Rania handed Sagesse the note.

"It says, '*Picked today. Please put into water immediately*

in the princess's sick room, for their scent is most precious'.
Oh, how lovely!"

"I think the scent is curative. You should have them by you in water for as long as the smell persists!" exclaimed Rania happily, thinking at last someone is taking proper care of the princess!

Sagesse smelled the flowers. "Oh yes, they do have a wonderful scent. Yes. Put them down here. I feel so much better, you know." And Rania put the flowers down near to Sagesse, who immediately bent down to smell them again and smiled broadly. Sagesse was hard put to explain why she felt so much better, but the smell of the flowers cheered her and she smiled several times.

On his third attempt at a cure, Kim resolved to sing to Sagesse. What mattered now was that Sagesse should get better and he didn't care anyway now if his cover was blown; he had everything he needed.

He had taken great pains to make sure of where her window was and a few days later he stood under it in the darkness, singing very softly in the hope that she'd catch some of the tune of the old folk song he had sung to her when they were children. Luckily, it happened that she came to the window and heard the sounds wafting upwards. She experienced such a sense of joy and wonder that she stayed watching the trees and the stars long after the singing had stopped. That evening Sagesse decided she was well enough to have her supper downstairs.

Kim on the other hand, as Distrell, had managed to get away unnoticed, only remarking to the guard on his way out of the main gate, that work had kept him later than usual.

* * *

The next morning, Kim, now in his own clothes, wearing comfortable shoes, his moustache shaven and no wig upon his head but a little, high hat, set out towards the palace. He wanted to arrive as a prince, but his heart was thumping with a fear that now he might easily be discovered by his father's men.

He was riding Modo, whom he had reclaimed that morning, so he would never be able to outrun his father's horses. His only disguise now was Modo – because his father's men did not know about the stalwart little donkey – and a scarf tied around Kim's neck, covering his chin.

As usual, he made his way through the most crowded places. Was that the most sensible thing to do? He wasn't sure. He had felt so alone and visible, even at night time, when he had come across Pelo, that crowds now seemed to be the best cover.

He and Modo plodded determinedly up the hill towards the palace, with Kim's ears out on stalks for any unexpected sounds. If any one of them saw him now, they *would* recognise him. Why had he been so stupid as to think he could get away with riding out as himself, without Kelin's hat – and on a donkey? Little Modo had no speed whatever; if he were chased by horses, they would catch him easily. Kim was tempting providence, thinking he had been lucky this far: surely providence would allow him this little step further?

Then, from down the hill came a terrifying, thundering sound, a sound that he had feared: the loud noise of horses' galloping hooves on the road.

"Get on Modo!" he yelled at the kindly, gentle donkey. "Go, go, go! Faster! Come on!" Modo picked up speed. In fact, sensing danger, Modo now moved faster than Kim had ever known him to move: sure-footed and uphill, he was suddenly trotting at a nice pace.

"Good Modo!" Kim was shouting. "Go it! Move like you've never moved before!" And Modo did just that. They were rounding the corner and the horses were rapidly catching them up.

"Keep going, Modo! We might make it!" The gate to the palace was near, but so were his father's soldiers. Would he get into the gate before the soldiers caught him? Kim was kicking poor Modo like mad to make him go quicker and they were almost at the gateway with the guard standing to attention. But the horses were almost upon them … just behind, rushing up … They were here … but so was the palace gateway!

The soldiers gathered round Kim so that Modo was unable to move.

"Stop! Stop, Prince Kim …" came a bellowing voice.

"Guard!" called Kim loudly. "These men are trying to stop me. But I have urgent business with your king." The guard came towards Kim, followed by another from the other side of the gateway. Both had pikes at the ready.

"You have business with King Ambab?" the first guard asked. "And who are these men?"

"They are King Demble's men from Strela. They want to stop me speaking to your king."

"And who are you?" asked the second guard.

"I am Prince Kim of Strela. I need to speak to King Ambab," Kim repeated.

Both guards now came out and stood between Kim and the soldiers. The first said loudly and clearly to the soldiers, "If you do anything to harm this young man, you are likely to create armed conflict with Beran soldiers. He is on Beran soil and as such he has the right to speak to our king, if the king wishes it."

The second guard now blew a horn and a messenger came, who was immediately sent back with one message for King Ambab and another for further soldiers to be brought to the main palace gates.

The messenger returned a minute later with the king's answer that he wished to see the prince, but that King Demble's soldiers must remain outside the gates. Further, well-armed soldiers arrived at the gateway to escort Kim to the king and to make sure the Strelan soldiers stayed outside the gates.

Meanwhile, during all this kerfuffle, Kim had managed to drop a letter into the roadway. It was later picked up by one of King Ambab's servants and found to contain a note from a certain Distrell. It said that the seemingly faithful employee, Distrell, had been forced to leave suddenly due to family problems in his homeland.

At the entrance to the palace, Kim handed Modo over

to the stable boy and entered the great hall where King Ambab came at once to meet him.

"How wonderful to see you! What on earth's going on? My people thought for a moment we were under attack!"

"Yes, they might well have thought that. It was I who was under attack. My father's men were trying to stop me seeing you."

"Why on earth would they do that?"

"Because I have some urgent and important information to give you and it does not speak well of my father. They would have forced me, as a prisoner, to be taken back to Strela. Your men saved me."

"My God, this is an outrage. Come, my dear, come in here and sit down. This is a shock." He led Prince Kim into a nearby sitting room.

"And all I had was my wonderful little donkey to help me escape them. He really galloped up the hill."

"Some kind of drink is in order, I think," King Ambab said after a moment. He said a few words to a servant and then turned back to Kim. "Come, we shall sit here and discuss your urgent matter."

This was a very different prince to the one King Ambab remembered – a slightly dirty, rather unkempt child, given to tempers, who was not afraid to answer back. That last quality had stood him in good stead, it seemed. Here was a young man who looked him in the eye and spoke to him like an equal.

They sat down now at the far end of a large sitting room, where anyone entering would not have heard what was being said at the other end of the room.

"I heard that you were travelling abroad ..." King Ambab said, looking over to Kim. "Your father didn't seem to know much when I last had occasion to speak to him."

"Well, I haven't written much. And my father – he seems to know about what I was doing and has been trying to prevent it. I did let them know I was all right. I went because my mother ..." Kim paused, anger welling up inside him remembering her last days. "She told me before she died that something terrible had happened which indirectly caused the death of my grandmother and directly caused the deaths of many people. And this thing was mainly brought about by my father and his brother Prince Callouste in a deal which they did together with you, King Ambab."

"Me?" He looked surprised. "Is this something I, personally, dealt with?"

"I think so. But I think you were not aware of what was going on, or of the theft of monies that should have gone to various communities in Strela. These monies were taken for the benefit solely of the two brothers, princes at the time, with the connivance of my grandfather, King Strearn, who had already amassed treasures easily worth the money they needed – and with you, possibly in ignorance ..."

"And how do you know all this? Believe this, I should say ..." asked King Ambab, taken aback by Kim's boldness. "Do you have proof?"

"I have three documents which prove what I say

beyond doubt." Kim was about to take them out when the door opened and Sagesse entered, excusing herself to Kim for interrupting, she went straight to her father.

"Father, did you know there are about fifty soldiers outside the palace gates? I think they're Strelan soldiers."

"Yes. And they have been stopped by Beran soldiers."

"They said it looked as if it was going to be a battle."

"It's all right now." There was a pause as the king looked at his daughter. "Aren't you going to say hullo to this person?" he exclaimed, indicating Kim.

Sagesse looked over to Kim and gasped. "Oh, my goodness! Kim! I didn't recognise you! You've changed … You look well. Was it you who brought the soldiers?"

"Hullo, Sagesse. Not exactly. I was just about to explain to your father …" Kim said to her, smiling. "But you've been ill, I hear."

"Oh, but I am almost better now. In fact, I feel very well indeed." And Sagesse was almost laughing. "I came in because I have something very urgent …" she turned to her father "to ask you, Father. And it's simply gone out of my head! Oh yes: will it be all right for me to tell Olmarlo to get the large carriage ready for all of us to go to Lake Daresna tomorrow? If we can get through the gates that is!"

"All …? What, us too?" asked King Ambab.

"Yes, if you want to! You too, Kim, if you would like."

"Yes, I would like that very much. Thank you."

"And while you're up and about like this," King Ambab said to his daughter, "tell Cook we have one extra for dinner. You'll stay, won't you Kim?"

"It would be a great pleasure. Thank you."

"You'll remain here with us, at the palace?"

"I already have a room in town," Kim said.

"Well, give it up. You're here as our guest!" King Ambab was beaming at him. "And now I want Kim to continue the story he was telling me. If you want to talk to him, you'll have to do so later."
Sagesse smiled.

"Yes," said Kim. "I would like to talk to you later."

"All right," she said. "We can meet under the veranda, before supper."

"See you there!" he said and Sagesse was off, out of the room.

"I was about to show you my documents," Kim said to King Ambab. "But I think first it would make more sense to tell you the whole story and then you can understand why the documents are so important."

So, Kim recounted to King Ambab as much of his story as was relevant. He said how he needed to find out the truth of what his mother had told him, no matter where it led, no matter what it took to find out. Finding this truth had become the whole purpose of his life, without which all other things, his friendships and family, could have no real meaning. He told him about Camdovin and his change of name and about the report he'd written.

At last Kim pulled out the three documents he had taken from King Ambab's own accounts library.

"And these three prove the truth of Camdovin's words," Kim said, handing them over to King Ambab.

When the king had finished reading them, he said

simply, "If I had seen these, I would have done something. The person in charge – I think it was, yes, it must have been someone named Malnir. He was sacked. We got rid of him because he hid the fact that another company had stolen funds. That was one I found out about. I also had suspicions that this man, Malnir, was in league with the company involved, but it was never proven. What you've given me here, I simply never knew at all."

"Camdovin heard them say they'd bribed your chief accountant."

"Listen. We must decide what to do about this. I'm guilty in that I should have known about it."

"But it was deliberately hidden from you!"

"All the same, it's my responsibility to know about these things. We should have sacked that scoundrel years earlier!" Ambab stopped and thought for a while. He got up and wandered towards the large windows which gave onto a well-kept part of the garden. "I'm trying to think how we can bring this, so to speak, to a conclusion," he said, eventually. "First, let me ring the bell for some lunch. We can continue on without disturbance, and it's a good excuse for me to get out of doing some extremely boring jobs!"

After lunch had been brought to the vast room and they had eaten, the king went on, "What I think would be feasible," he drained a glass of wine, "is if I write a letter to both Callouste and Demble stating that three important documents have come to my attention – I certainly won't say how or why – proving that they robbed the people of Strela of large sums of money, causing widespread contamination to the water and depriving many of their lives; many died, you said ..."

"Yes, many thousands, causing a curse to be put on the Strelan royal family amongst other things ... and people close to them, as well as many thousands of the people of Strela."

"I'll insist they make amends, otherwise I'll have these documents made known to the general public."

"That's good! And you should also tell them that other powerful people have seen the documents – you don't have to say who – and if anything happens to you, they will immediately make this whole thing public."

"Yes. I shall give it a while before I write. Say two or three months. You'll have a chance to be home and settled by then."

"And I'll tell Camdovin what you intend to do. Also, I think the King of Memarn will be interested," said Kim.

"I might remind Demble," said King Ambab, "that if his people know all this, they would probably kill him. So, he'll have to decide."

* * *

Later that day, Kim waited for Sagesse under the veranda. When she arrived, he kissed her hand formally.

"I can't tell you how happy I am to see you looking well," he said to her.

"And you ... The last time I saw you, I don't think you were that well ..."

"No ... in more ways than one. And of course, my

mother had just died. But I am better now. Come," Kim said to her and he led the way, through the trees and grass to the old, hollow oak.

"We played here when we were children. And I once said to you that if you ever needed my assistance in anything, large or small, you were to call upon me. I say it again to you," he spoke in a rather formal way because he felt so much love for her that he didn't know how to express it and, at the same time, he didn't want to burden her with it. And when he saw her eyes he knew, without any doubt, that he had been carrying her around with him all this time; for the talisman that Tiésa had given to him, in the form of a woman's face, showed none other than Sagesse herself. And he knew that he no longer had need of the talisman or even to ride a donkey, because having found his heart's desire he could ride on a horse if he wanted to – though he had grown so fond of the stately travel of his little donkey, Modo, that he doubted he would ever give him up.

He kissed her hand again and she realised it was he who had cured her; she knew that she would visit him and that whatever else happened to them they would always remain the closest of friends.

Then Sagesse said, "Thank you for what you have done for me, and I will look forward to coming to Strela to see you and your sister." The two of them walked together, slowly back through the garden, with Kim deeply thankful that the curse was now broken.

Chapter 18
RETURN TO KOREMINE

When Kim arrived back at Koremine Castle, he adopted a stance of total innocence with his father. They both ignored the fact that Kim had almost been captured by his father's men. Kim would pretend he hadn't noticed the soldiers searching for him and trying to stop him. Yes, he'd had an interesting time, when asked.

"How did you live?" asked King Demble.

"Oh, doing this and that …" Kim was as vague as he could be.

"Odd jobs? What did they think of a prince doing odd jobs?" the king naively asked.

"They didn't know I was a prince."

"They must have thought something of your magnificent horse, Plarus."

"But Plarus was stolen from me by border guards."

"And were you living in the countryside?" asked the king.

"Most of the time," Kim lied. "I did go to visit King Ambab." He wanted to give his father a reason for General Misot and the army's failing to find him.

"So you were not in any of the main towns at all?"

Clearly, King Demble decided, his thinking had been all wrong about his son; maybe there had been nothing to fear from him after all and making General Misot search for him had been a costly mistake. Fortunately for Kim, General Misot had been so angry and ashamed at his failure to capture Kim at the gates of Vocimere Palace that he had only reported it back to King Demble in a very unclear way. "We missed him by just a few minutes. But I don't think he knew we were following him," he added, lying to save his skin from the king's wrath.

Pala was, of course, overjoyed to see her brother safe and sound.

"Thank God you're here, at last! Why did it take you so long?" she cried when, after seeing him from a window, she rushed out to meet him, flinging her arms around him almost before he had time to get off poor Modo. "And who's this sweet little donkey? Where's Plarus?" The questions tumbled from her long before Kim had time to answer. "I got a few letters from you, but why didn't you give me an address so that I could answer?" And then: "You look so different!"

As Kim embraced his sister it was clear to him that Pala was no longer quiet and taciturn; it seemed she had grown more graceful, more serious and, with her brother unexpectedly returned, more talkative than ever before.

"What have you been doing all this time?" Kim asked as they sat in his room, with him feeling a bit guilty that his travels had prevented him from keeping up with her news. "Have you been studying hard?"

"Yes, I have. And also helping the poor people in the countryside, and …. and …" she stuttered.

"And what?" Kim asked, laughing. He could immediately see that although he had not said a word to her about the curse and the result of his searches, Pala was obviously feeling the benefits of his success. At last, as in contrast with the morose, angry, silent girl he had left behind at Koremine Castle, Pala had changed into a healthy, happy person, full of hope.

"And …" Pala went on, "I did something terrible!" She was now looking stricken with remorse.

"What was that?" asked Kim, with a fairly clear idea of what it might have been.

"I told Father that you were trying to find a stranger …. I am so sorry! He wanted to have a party … Imagine! A month after Mother had died, a week or so after you had gone. I just let rip at him and said I didn't want a party: I was sad because of Mother and because you had gone away looking for some stranger who knew something important. I think I wanted to shock him …"

"And did you?"

"Have the party? No!"

"No, I mean did you shock him?" asked Kim.

"Oh, yes, I think I did. Anyway, he stopped going on at me."

"And you know what he did then?"

"No. What?" asked Pala, surprised.

"He organised men to come and look for me. His soldiers. I saw them in Memarn and in Beran," he said.

"Eventually they almost caught me in Beran, when I was going into the palace."

"Oh, no! My God! But how did you escape them?" she exclaimed

"Well, the first time I saw them, they were about ten of them, all riding down the street, towards me in Trasimid. Luckily, I had an old hat on, which practically covered my face …" And Kim told Pala about hiding behind the great wooden door for an hour until the men had gone away. He praised the virtues of the large hat that Kelin had given him which had hidden his face and the benefits of riding a donkey instead of a horse; and eventually they laughed about it and Pala's mind was eased.

Soon after his return, Kim contacted his friend Cal. He swore him to secrecy as they walked along the outskirts of Koremine Town, and then he was able to tell him most of what had happened on his search.

"How come those men of your father's didn't find you? From what you say they were all over Trasimid," asked Cal. "Weren't you scared? I would have been!"

"I was. Especially the first time I saw them, riding down the street all in a bunch like that. Terrified." And he told Cal about Kelin's hat.

"He should be in prison! Your father! To conspire to commit – what? Mass murder? So, what will happen when King Ambab writes his letter to King Demble? What's to be done?"

"It's a good question," answered Kim. "I think he'll have to abdicate – or else be torn apart by his suffering people!"

"And then you'll be king! What will you do with him and your uncle? Put them in prison? You can't do that."

"I'll have to do something similar," said Kim. "Maybe not exactly prison, but some kind of house arrest for him and his horrible wife! The same for my uncle Callouste. That is, if they go quietly."

"Well let's hope they do go quietly," said Cal, looking doubtful.

"I hope so too," answered Kim, as they continued their walk.

* * *

When, after three months, King Ambab wrote his letter to King Demble, giving details of all his and his brother's crimes, threatening to publicise across many lands their evil deeds so that people from different countries would be free to take their revenge, King Demble knew that Kim and his mother, Queen Donata, had irrevocably won in their mission.

His immediate response was to start shouting. At everyone. First, he caught Pala at breakfast and accused her.

"It was you, wasn't it, who knew all about what Kim was doing? Was it you who planned it?"

Poor Pala. She didn't know what to say, except, "No, no! I didn't know anything about it all. I didn't even know where Kim was ..." She tried not to burst into tears and run upstairs to her room, but sat there stoically, eating the rest of her breakfast in silence.

The next person who got it was the old and trusted servant, Sen, who had been at the palace from his youth.

"Was it you?" shouted King Demble. "You and the queen who put my son up to this?"

"Up to what, Your Majesty?" asked the ever-polite servant.

"You know very well! Don't pretend to me that you are ignorant of what's been going on behind my back. Don't pretend to me!" the king repeated.

Then it was the stable boy and later even General Misot who got a bawling out for being in the wrong place at the wrong time.

"You could have stopped him!" the king shouted. "You were nearly there! You could have caught him, but you let him pass. Did he bribe you?"

"Your Majesty," the general's voice became unnaturally quiet, as he really didn't like being shouted at or, indeed, countered in any way at all. It was he himself who had always been in the position of doing the shouting and making the decisions. "We were prevented from capturing your son because King Ambab's men came out in force. With our fifty soldiers, we would have had to do battle against what could have become a thousand of King Ambab's men. Such a thing was never in my brief and I decided we would have no chance of success in that situation. So, yes, we backed down. The only sensible decision to take."

"A wrong decision!" King Demble would not give up. "I am ruined because of this …"

"Another decision I have made," continued the

imperturbable general quietly, "is that I no longer wish to be in your service." With that the general turned and left the room with the king standing speechless.

King Demble's outburst at Kim was, understandably, the most violent of all. He shouted, he ranted, he raved and eventually threatened the wrath of Satan to fall upon Kim.

"If you do not get King Ambab to retract his letter – take every word of it back – I shall wage war on him."

"I cannot do that, Father." Kim was as polite as possible; after all, it was not a nice thing to watch his father in defeat. "As I understand it, if you don't capitulate and give up the throne, King Ambab will make public your crimes to all the countries around and to all those who have suffered because of you."

By this time King Demble was shouting again. "How dare you go against your own father in this! You want the crown for yourself! You are nothing but a disloyal son bent on gaining the crown!" He stopped to catch his breath.

"All I care about," said Kim, "is that there is a person on the Strelan throne who is honest and kind to his people and who does not cause them starvation, contamination and illness deliberately. Such a person is not a leader, he is a despot. Anyone who rules this country must take care of the people in it."

King Ambab had stipulated in his letter that King Demble should abdicate immediately and hand over all reins of office to the next in line to the throne whom, he believed, would probably be Prince Kim (although he said nothing to suggest that he'd had any conversation with Kim). The letter was strong and decisive and gave no sign as to where King Ambab had got his information. The next king or queen should be the one to decide on his and his brother's punishment.

Naturally, Kim had been mulling this over for the months between his return and King Ambab's letter and, after discussions with Pala and Cal, they had all agreed that both his father and Prince Callouste should remain in "house arrest" at specific and separate locations: two country houses where they must stay at all times. There would not be any public explanation about their confinement, but they would have no access to any communication, monies, army personnel or power of any kind. It would be made known to the general public that the two had collaborated in a serious crime.

And, so it happened. Kim became king and the two evil brothers were sent away in shame – though most people could only guess why.

A few months after Kim's accession to the throne he and Sagesse were betrothed – her mother, Queen Flura, having not the power to prevent her marrying a king, and one whom her husband seemed to admire beyond measure.

As king, Kim sorted through the ministers, weeding out the bad ones and finding good ones. He appointed Cal as "the king's special adviser" and ruled the kingdom wisely and generously.

With Lullam now freed from jail and working happily at Ardair, there were visits to Koremine Castle from

Camdovin and Atrell and their children, including the young Alman, who formed a strong attachment to Pala. Alman came back to see her on several occasions and eventually they married.

Kelin also came with his family and Tiésa even visited once (though she didn't like travelling), taking back her talisman and pronouncing her young friend well settled.

* * *

"And what was the most frightening part of your whole journey?" asked Sagesse, as she, Kim and Cal sat around one evening after supper. "Was it when the robbers attacked you? Or when your father's men were coming down the busy main Trasimid road towards you and you had to hide?" They all laughed, imagining their new young king pulling Kelin's old hat well down over his eyes.

"Or being thrown into prison?" put in Cal, more seriously. "That must have been frightening." Kim nodded his assent, gravely.

"Or all those soldiers coming after you, just before you reached the palace gates. Terrifying," Sagesse said. "The noise of that inside the palace was weird, because it was like a quiet rumble that just got louder and louder and louder; and it wasn't really recognisable as horses' hooves, just a rumbling and a shaking of everything."

"That was truly frightening indeed. I thought I wouldn't make it. I can't think why I didn't stay in my disguise – or at least keep on Kelin's hat. That was mad.

But almost the scariest thing of all was somehow also really creepy; and that was late at night, when I was going to my room from the palace in my full disguise as Distrell, along a lonely road. I saw a man coming straight towards me and it was Pelo."

"Pelo? Who's that?" questioned Cal.

"Another of my father's men. Pelo. He came towards me and when I saw who it was, I was praying he wouldn't recognise me. And then he stopped me and asked me if I knew some road or other, so I said (in my funny voice) that I wasn't from the area and I knew that if I ran, I wouldn't have a chance anyway with the bits of wood in my shoes. I got round the corner, out of sight, and took out the bits of wood and ran for it. And then he arrived at the corner. If he'd have walked past my tree, I'm sure he would have known I was there because of the sound of my heartbeat: it was thumping. Anyway, thank God he gave up." Kim looked serious for a moment longer. "Well, all that's over now ..." and he laughed.

"And who was the most helpful of all your friends?" asked Cal, after a moment. "I mean, was it Tiésa or Kelin or Camdovin, or I don't know – Habama, King Ambab – who?"

"That's a difficult one." Kim got up and walked about for a moment. "They were all important in their own way," he went on. "I wouldn't have been able to do it without them. Not one of them." He sat down again. "Perhaps it was someone you didn't mention." He smiled. "A 'person' who kept me company all the way – or most of it, anyway; who did everything I asked and made no fuss whatever, and who, just as I was getting near Vocimere Palace, with fifty soldiers chasing me, made the most stupendous effort of all. It was little Modo, who rushed up that hill in a way you would never believe of a donkey; he galloped when I told him to! If donkeys can gallop, that is."

THE END